HERBAL ELIXIRS

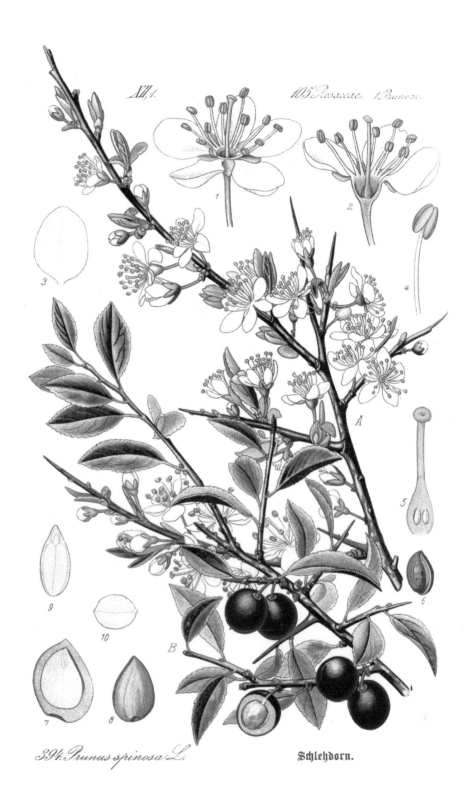

XII,1.   105.*Rosaceae. 1.*Pruneae.*

394.*Prunus spinosa L.*   Schlehdorn.

HERBAL ELIXIRS

A Guide to Making Your Own Medicinal Drinks

Sue Mullett and Jade Harris

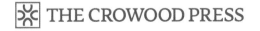 THE CROWOOD PRESS

First published in 2021 by
The Crowood Press Ltd
Ramsbury, Marlborough
Wiltshire SN8 2HR

enquiries@crowood.com

www.crowood.com

British Library Cataloguing-in-Publication Data
A catalogue record for this book is available from the British Library.

ISBN 978 1 78500 886 3

Acknowledgements
We would like to express our heartfelt thanks to Rob Mullett for his help and advice.

The image on page 10 is from Cécily Lucas, Nicolas Barnich and Hang Thi Thu Nguyen - Microbiota, Inflammation and Colorectal Cancer, Int. J. Mol. Sci. 2017, 18(6), 1310; doi:10.3390/ijms18061310.

Disclaimer
The authors and the publisher do not accept any responsibility in any manner whatsoever for any error or omission, or any loss, damage, injury, adverse outcome, or liability of any kind incurred as a result of the use of any of the information contained in this book, or reliance upon it.

Typeset by Catherine Williams, Chapter One Book Production

Cover design by Blue Sunflower Creative

Printed and bound in India by Parksons Graphics

Contents

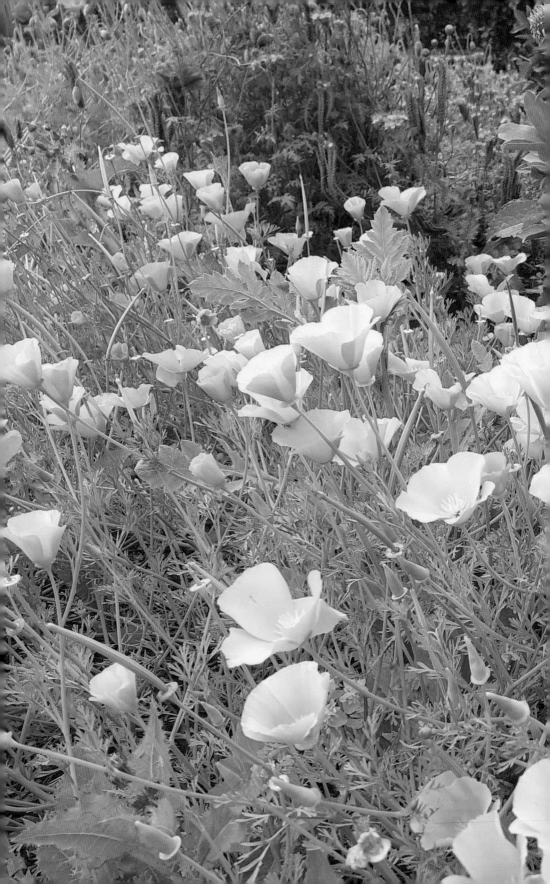

Part 1
History

Introduction

The rapid modernization of the last century brought many undeniable benefits, but it was also accompanied by a growing dislocation from the natural environment and many traditional practices. This book explores the rich history of medicinal alcohol in Europe, which has largely been obscured by modern institutional medicine and a drinks industry that tends to promote hedonistic over-indulgence.

We will share our knowledge and skills to allow you to produce your own herbal drinks, tinctures, syrups, and alcohol. Drawing on our own experience of blending the skills of the herbalist and distiller in our small botanical gin distillery in the historic city of Bath, we will talk you through how to source and preserve your herbs, distil your base alcohol, prepare herbal tinctures, make syrups, and, finally, blend and store your creations. In the process, we hope to bring you more in tune with the amazing variety of medicinal plants that are to be found in our hedgerows and fields, and to inspire you to create your very own delicious blends.

What Are Herbal Elixirs?

The inspiration behind this book is the range of herbal elixirs that we produce in our small distillery in Bath. Herbal elixirs are alcoholic drinks with medicinal properties, made by blending different herbs and syrups together with alcohol. Ours are influenced by the use of herbal drinks throughout history, not only as recreational drinks but also as beverages that offer benefits to health. All too often, the modern conception of alcoholic drinks associates them only with pleasure and indulgence, yet this view overshadows a far more complex tradition. Alcohol has a unique set of

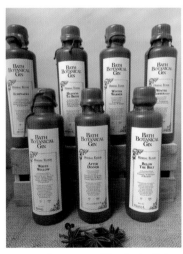

A range of herbal elixirs.

properties that make it an ideal solvent to extract and preserve the active chemical constituents of herbs. These qualities have led to a long association between distillation and herbal medicine.

The idea of medicinal spirits drunk both for pleasure and for health might seem too good to be true to modern ears. However, this has arguably been their dominant form in Europe until relatively recently, from the digestive tonics made by the Ancient Romans infusing herbs into wine, to the classic European aperitifs and digestifs of the nineteenth century. There is a particularly long history of alcoholic drinks created to enjoy before and after meals, to stimulate the appetite, help with digestion, and maintain a healthy body – not to mention adding a flavour of their own! Many popular drinks that are enjoyed today, such as Aperol and Cinzano, still fulfil a similar role, although arguably their medicinal properties are not necessarily their main appeal.

Guided by this tradition, we have designed our herbal elixirs by combining herbal tinctures with our self-produced gin to create alcoholic drinks that can provide therapeutic benefits when consumed responsibly. We have also added various syrups and sweeter herbs in order to create a pleasing flavour profile. As many practising medical herbalists discover, blends of herbal tinctures, although extremely useful therapeutically, cannot often be said to be pleasant-tasting. Indeed, such concoctions can be counterproductive as herbal remedies. Unlike the quick fix of modern pharmaceuticals, they need to be taken regularly for a number of weeks for their benefits to start to be effective. If a mixture does not taste good, it is less likely that someone will persist in their treatment. It was with this in mind that we started to design drinks that are both therapeutic and drinkable. Currently, it is impossible to find blends of tinctures on the market that have been blended for their therapeutic benefit, but can also be enjoyed as a delicious drink. It is this that has prompted the writing of this book, as we are keen to promote the use and enjoyment of herbs.

As with any alcoholic product, we advise you to consume our products responsibly, although they have a relatively low alcohol content in comparison with spirits such as whisky or rum. Our elixirs have been designed to be taken in small amounts before or after a meal. Consuming more than a small glass per day will not increase any therapeutic benefits and may, in fact, compromise the body's ability to absorb and process the herbal tinctures contained within.

The Authors

Sue Mullett is the founder of Bath Botanical Gin Distillery. She has a BSc in Western Medical Herbalism, and is a prolific raider of the hedgerows and fruit trees of the south-west of England.

Jade Harris developed an interest in ancient medicines whilst studying classics. She now works as an assistant in the distillery and in her spare time is a keen grower of unusual herbs.

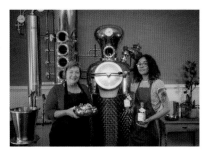

The authors: Jade Harris and Sue Mullett.

Together, we produce a range of gins and bitters in our beautiful copper still, using locally foraged herbs and fruits. Alongside our more conventional offerings, we also produce a range of herbal elixirs that have been inspired by traditional drinks produced across Europe. These drinks combine blends of herbs that are designed both to be delicious and, if consumed responsibly, to have therapeutic properties.

Our Ethos

Our book can be seen as a small part of a much wider trend known as the 'functional food movement'. This is based around a shift in the idea of food and drink as only providing 'fuel' for the body. Instead, food is seen as both fuel and medicine. The movement has grown out of attempts to understand the changes in the types of illness that are most common across the Western world.

The developments in modern medical care have been nothing short of miraculous. They have raised life expectancy and lowered the infant mortality rate significantly, through a mixture of radical breakthroughs in surgical techniques, effective use of vaccinations to control and even eradicate formerly dangerous diseases, the development of antibiotics to control infection, and drugs that help alleviate the symptoms of chronic diseases. However, although it has been possible to treat and control many of the diseases that were formerly prolific, there has been a rise in the incidence of a different set of diseases and chronic conditions, including obesity, diabetes and asthma. Despite its many successes, modern medicine seems to be fighting a losing battle against these health issues. This apparent failure has prompted a lot of soul-searching and research. As a result, a new picture of the human body has emerged, with a call for a more holistic approach to health care, and a focus on the types of food and drink that we consume.

Typically, the body of the individual has been envisaged as a closed unit, separate and genetically distinct from the world outside. Microorganisms such as bacteria and fungi have been seen as a threat to this unit, leading to a concerted effort to eliminate them, not only from the body but also from our homes, food and drink. Whilst it is true that microorganisms can and do cause serious illness, the effort to cleanse ourselves and our environment has brought negative health impacts of its own. This is due to the misconception of the body as a closed unit containing cells only with the individual's unique genetic code. In fact, there is evidence to show that 'only about half the cells in our bodies contain a "human genome"' (Scott, 2017). The rest are made up of vast microbial networks, which, far from harming the body, actually play an essential role in its healthy function. Perhaps the most significant concentration of these essential microbial communities is in the gut, where they are collectively known as the microbiome, or the microbiota.

Although we might think of the gut and its health as being central only to the uptake of food, in truth its role is much more varied and complex. First, it forms an essential part of the immune system – indeed, it accounts for around two-thirds of it – making it key to a better understanding and treatment of autoimmune disorders that relate to inflammation in the body. It has also been linked to mental health, giving a new meaning to the phrase 'thinking with your stomach'. As Scott Anderson writes in his fascinating exploration of the links between the brain and the gut, *The Psychobiotic Revolution*, 'for good health, including good mental health, the food you eat needs to be good for you *and* your microbiota'.

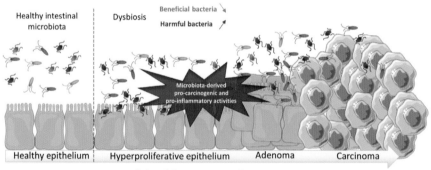

Bacteria in the human intestine (Lucas et al, 2017).

The idea that, through the bacteria in our gut, food affects our health is the basis of the functional food movement. These concepts can be seen in the work of herbalists and nutritionists, who have begun to see the diet as a therapeutic tool. Dietary recommendations and nutritional supplements are now well understood and used widely throughout the Western world. Unfortunately, however, the benefits of alcoholic extractions of herbs are less well understood, and their use is less common. The main reason for this is a fear of the misuse of alcohol, which has led to the strict regulations that govern its manufacture and sale. For example, in the European Union, very complex regulations control the claims that can be made for various herbal products and nutritional supplements. In the United Kingdom, even products containing a little as 0.25% of alcohol have specific labelling requirements, including a ban on any claim of therapeutic uses or health benefits. This is why you will not see any herbal alcoholic drinks making such claims or even explaining the traditional use of herbs. In contrast, you will notice that teas using similar mixtures of herbs are allowed to list their therapeutic effects and the packaging will often feature information about the uses of the relevant herbs.

Our hope is that, as the functional food movement continues to take off, and as doctors begin to integrate herbs, nutrition and lifestyle changes into health practice, qualified individuals will be able to educate consumers about the vast historical benefits and uses of herbs that have helped humans survive long enough to be here today. It should then be possible to sell delicious herbal elixirs, with their potential health benefits clearly stated on the label.

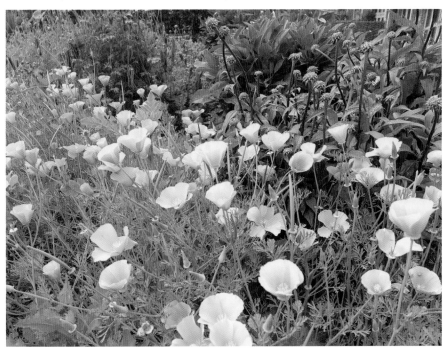

Herb garden with Californian poppies and purple cone flowers (Echinacea).

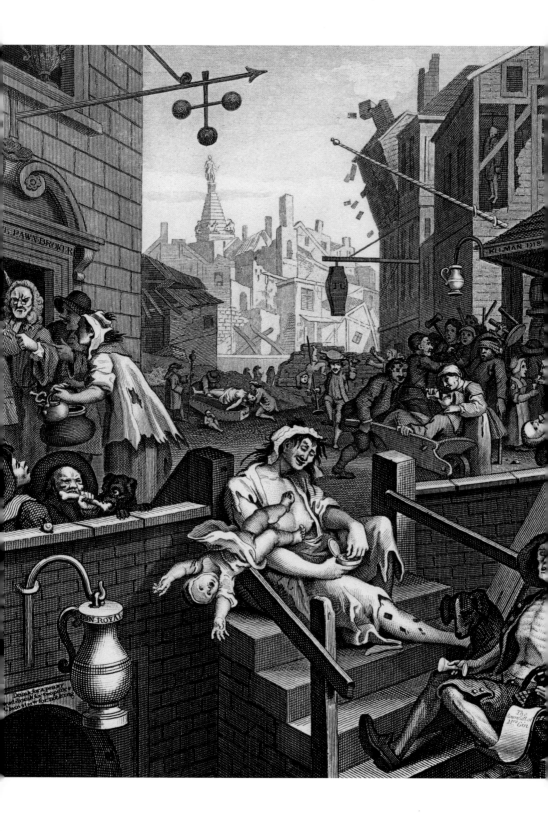

1

The History of Herbal Drinks

Humanity's relationship with alcohol and fermentation stretches back as far as written records go. Reconnecting with this past provides an interesting contrast with the current perception and uses of alcohol. In the past, the production of alcohol and the uses of fermentation were focused far more on the therapeutic and preservative than on the purely recreational. We hope that through engaging with the history of alcohol we will be able to shift attitudes and bring about a fundamental rethink that puts the medicinal possibilities of alcoholic drinks firmly back on the table.

Medical school in Salerno, Italy, in the Middle Ages – the most prestigious and innovative medical school of its time; where medicine first became a profession and alcohol was distilled for solely medicinal usage.

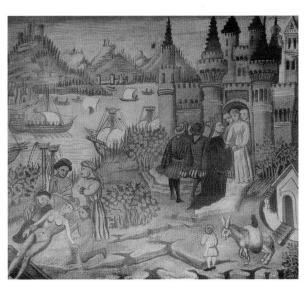

As this book deals primarily with Western medical traditions, our brief historical sketch will focus predominantly on Europe, the Middle East and northern Africa. It is worth noting, however, that these are far from the only places with a rich history relating to alcohol and distillation. There were large civilizations across the globe, from North and South America to Asia, that easily rivalled or surpassed those within and around Europe in terms of their own cultural practices regarding the use of alcohol.

Historic Timeline

Prehistory
Prehistory refers to the time before written records.

Fermentation is a process that is continually occurring in the natural world. As such, it is impossible to pinpoint the exact time when it began to be harnessed by humans. It is likely that it would first have been observed tens of thousands of years ago, in the natural fermentation of fallen fruit. Archaeological evidence of Stone Age beer jugs indicates that the use of fermentation to produce alcoholic drinks existed as early as Neolithic times, some ten thousand years ago. Unfortunately, it is not possible to determine from these remains the way in which alcoholic drinks were being used – did they play a role in drunken antics or were they part of a more complicated cultural practice?

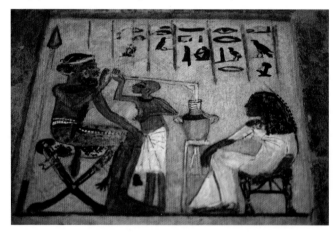

Pouring out of beer. An Egyptian hieroglyph showing that fermentation was an important part of life as beer was commonly drunk.

It is only much later that a more detailed picture of the uses of alcohol emerges, through early written records from ancient societies. For example, Egyptian pictographs dating back to 4000 BC depict not only the preparation and consumption of wine but also show the different way in which the people enjoyed it. Studies show that the Ancient Egyptians indulged in the intoxicating effects of alcohol recreationally, not unlike today. However, this civilization also provides some of the earliest evidence of the combining of medicinal herbs and alcohol. The tomb of an early Egyptian pharaoh, Scorpian I, contained numerous jars that, when analysed, revealed a number of medicinal herbs mixed with wine.

The lack of written and archaeological evidence from this period means that it is difficult to make any assumptions about attitudes towards alcohol. However, given the variety of cultures and societies that would have existed, it is safe to assume that the beginnings of the human relationship with alcohol was not exclusively a dysfunctional one.

Ancient History

This covers the period between 3000 BC and 500 AD, from the beginnings of writing and recorded history until the fall of the Western Roman Empire.

The extensive literature of the Greek and Roman Empire indicates an increasingly complex relationship with alcohol and its therapeutic uses. Even the Gods themselves could not help but get involved and, through Dionysus and Bacchus, alcohol even had its own divine representation. At this point, despite the advances in science and technology, the art of distillation had yet to be perfected on a large scale and was not in common usage. As a result, alcohol was produced and consumed in the form of a variety of wines and beers. Like the Egyptians before them, the Romans used wine not only used for recreation but also frequently as a component of ancient medicine.

The beginnings of many modern disciplines can be traced back to the work of Ancient Greek philosophers. Maths and science began to take forms that are familiar today, through the work of thinkers such as Aristotle and Pythagoras. There were significant developments in medicine, too, and chief among the names that remain strongly connected to the Western medical tradition is Hippocrates. His ethical framework for the practice of medicine is still alive and well in the form of the Hippocratic Oath, which is taken by medical professionals across the globe. Within his therapeutic practices, it is clear that the negative views on the health impacts of alcohol had not yet taken hold. Indeed, he recommends the use of a variety of therapeutic herbs

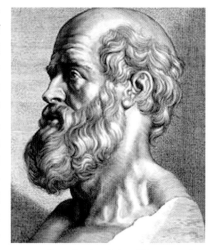

Greek physician Hippocrates (460–370 BC) was the founder a medical school on the island of Kos. He is often referred to as the 'father of modern medicine'.

soaked in wines as remedies for a number of ailments. One example, as a relief from digestive troubles and specifically to treat intestinal parasites, is white wine infused with wormwood. It is interesting to note that the mixture of wine and wormwood continues today in vermouth, although it is accompanied by a number of other herbs and roots.

Dioscorides, a physician in the Roman army, was another highly influential figure, although his work is considerably less well known than that of his predecessor. Dioscorides used his experience of travelling around Europe with the army to collect and record local uses of different herbs in remedies for a variety of conditions. He gathered together this knowledge into a vast five-volume medical textbook that was highly valued throughout Europe and the Middle East and was still in use centuries later. Like Hippocrates, he also suggested the use of wine both as a solvent and as a preservative for herbal remedies.

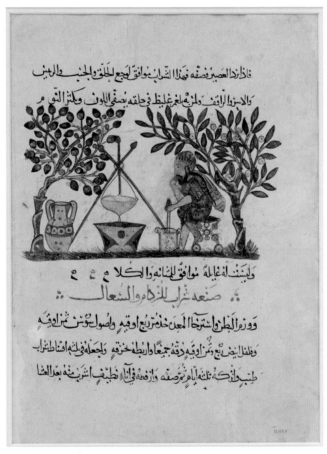

Dioscorides' *Materis Medica*, a 1334 text in Arabic
describing the medicinal features of cumin and dill.

The Middle Ages

This is considered to be the period, dating from the fall of the Roman Empire until the fifteenth century.

The decline of the Roman Empire brought with it the rise of religion as an important site of both political power and scientific innovation. The relationship between religion and science has not been without conflict and to the modern mind the two can often be thought of as mutually exclusive. This has not always been the case. Islamic scholars in the Middle East became one of the primary driving forces behind science and innovation at this time; among their many achievements was the refinement of the practice of distillation. Whilst simple forms of distillation were no doubt occurring across the globe prior to this, it was the combination of metal-working skills, a knowledge of the materials and an understanding of the physics behind distillation that led to the invention of the copper alembic still. It is a design that is still in use today – testament to the ingenuity and skill of its inventors.

It was not only the art of distillation that advanced in this period but also the bank of medical knowledge. A good example can be found in the work of Islamic Scholar Ibn Sina, a Persian philosopher, mathematician and poet, who among his many pursuits managed to find the time to write two medical texts: *The Book of Healing* and *The Canon of Medicine*. The latter was a hug medical encyclopaedia that became a key text and was used in medical schools until the seventeenth century.

The invention of the alembic still meant that distilled alcohol became widely available across Europe and the Middle East for the first time. It was quickly discovered that the capacity of alcohol to extract and preserve the active elements of herbs was greatly increased in line with the strength of the alcoholic solutions. It is no doubt due to the widespread use of distilled alcohol in medicine that it was often referred to as *aqua vita*, or 'water of life'. These developments brought with them an increasing professionalization of medical and pharmacological practices. As the body of medical knowledge and texts grew, so did the number of medical schools, and apothecaries became an increasingly common sight on the streets. However, access to this increasing fund of knowledge was still restricted to a relatively small and privileged group, centred around religious institutions such as monasteries.

Renaissance

Overlapping with the Middle Ages, the Renaissance is considered to start with the fall of Constantinople in 1453.

The two central influencing factors of this period were the growth in the influence and spread of monasteries throughout Europe and the beginnings of colonization, which brought with it access to many new herbs and spices. Although there had been trade in spices between European and Asian countries previously, the scale and scope of the operations increased significantly over this period. Previously, those who were engaged in preparing medicines were dealing directly with Arab traders, who worked on a comparatively small scale and were therefore having to sell at very high prices. Indeed, some spices cost more than gold. With the opening up of international trade routes, the apothecaries could buy from larger companies such as the Dutch East Indies and the British East India. These powerful and influential enterprises had an impressive number of ships at their disposal and, with the exploitation of resources imposed through colonization, were able to sell their products in much greater quantities and at much lower prices.

As a result of different products becoming more readily available, bringing new flavours with them, herbal medicinal drinks began to shift from being solely for therapeutic purposes into being enjoyed for their taste as well.

Early Modernity
1600–1850

During this period, there was an acceleration in the changes and advancements in society, technology, science, arts and trade. At the beginning of the seventeenth century, distillation was increasing in terms of scale and commercialization.

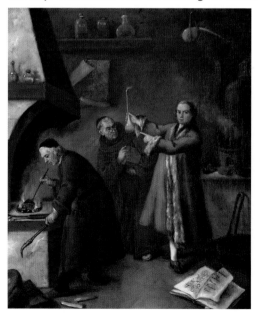

Previously, many herbal drinks had been made on a small scale, and there was a great deal of local variation. As time went on, they began to be mass-produced, with many losing their links with medicine and becoming seen primarily as substances that were to be consumed for the purpose of intoxication.

The Alchemists by Pietro Longhi, 1757. Alchemists improved distillation techniques in their quest to find a panacea for all common ills and to transform base metals into gold.

Gin is the perfect example of a spirit that was originally designed to be used as a medicine and later became a popular mass-produced drink. The central ingredient of gin, juniper berries, had been found to be useful in the treatment of the fevers and tropical diseases suffered by the Dutch as they colonized the East Indies. Gin was originally sold in pharmacies but, by the middle of the eighteenth century, it was being mass-produced in Holland and had been exported to Britain. There, its medicinal properties seem to have been forgotten and it was increasingly used as an intoxicant. Widespread excessive alcohol consumption became a serious social problem and the harmful effects of cheap spirits such as gin are believed to have put the very fabric of British society in danger. Written and pictorial records of the time show the debauchery associated with gin bars across the country and especially in the capital, London. Medical professionals, such as the members of the Royal College of Physicians, began to voice their concerns about the 'pernicious and growing use of spirituous liquors' and their effects upon individuals and society. A number of petitions were submitted to parliament to seek legislation to curb the misuse of alcoholic drinks.

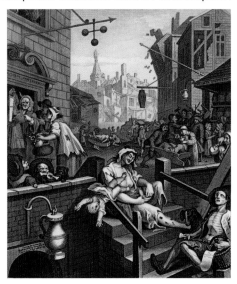

Gin Lane: 1751 engraving by Hogarth, depicting the evils of alcohol consumption in London during the 'gin craze'.

Modern Times
1850 to present day

Clearly, through history a number of factors have influenced the ways in which society perceives and uses alcohol: the technology affecting the strength and speed at which it can be produced, the knowledge of the pharmacological effects of certain herbs, and the institutions that control this knowledge and/or the means of production. Attitudes towards alcohol and its predominant forms in the modern era indicate that many of the same influences are still relevant, either directly or through the cultural legacy that they have left behind.

Perhaps the clearest influences in the modern drinks industry are commercialization and mechanization. The trend of mass-producing popular medicinal spirits such as gin for recreational consumption has continued and indeed increased. The turn of the century brought with it many of the well-known brands of herbal aperitifs and digestifs that still exist today, such as vermouth and Amer Picon. These drinks were often based on herbal recipes developed by monks across Europe, who in turn had been influenced by Middle Eastern medical scholars. As time has gone by, the medicinal roots of these recipes and drinks have largely been forgotten. Alcohol is perceived less as the 'water of life' than as a negative element in terms of personal health.

The demonization of alcohol can also be traced back to the religious Protestant ideals of temperance, which were behind the calls for prohibition in the United States in the 1920s and 1930s. This was coupled with the rise of a pharmaceutical industry that preferred to extract and patent the active elements of herbs, and administer the doses in forms that do not use alcohol, such as pills and injections. As a result, the role of alcohol as a key substance within medicine has largely been forgotten.

This book will show you the ways in which alcohol can be produced and how it can be used to extract and preserve herbs. It will guide you through the common herbs that can be found in Northern Europe and their therapeutic uses. Lastly, it will provide you with recipes to create your own modern herbal elixirs, inspired by a long tradition of herbal drinks.

2

Commercially Available Herbal Drinks

There are a number of traditional herb-based alcoholic beverages that remain on the market today, although often their medical origins are no longer widely known. In this section we will be exploring some of these drinks, their ingredients and a little about their history. The recipe for some remains a closely guarded secret, but fortunately this is not always the case.

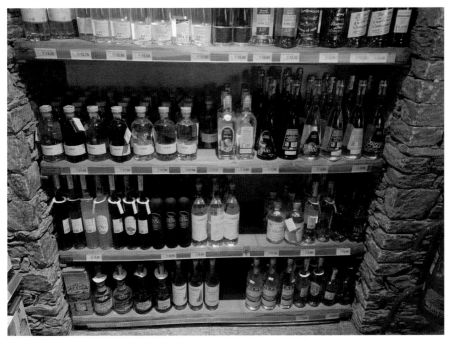

The large range of herbal drinks available in Italian supermarkets in 2020.

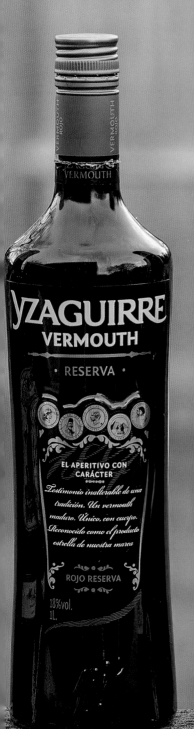
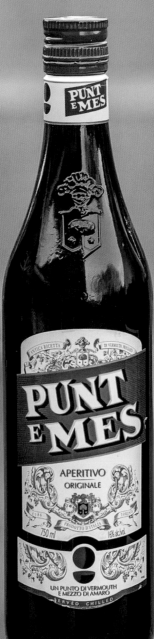
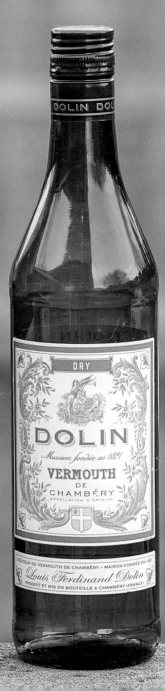

These drinks can be loosely divided into three categories. First, there are herbal aperitifs. These are relatively weak, with an alcohol content of between 15 and 20%, which have been designed to help cleanse the palate and improve digestion using combinations of bitter-tasting herbs. They are traditionally served before a meal in a small glass. Second, there are the digestifs, which are of a similar strength and are served in a similar style. However, they are designed to be consumed after a meal is eaten, to prevent indigestion, contain aromatic herbs such as mint and fennel, and are often sweetened. Finally, there are herbal spirits such as absinthe, which are much stronger, at around 40%. Care should be taken to avoid overconsumption of herbal spirits.

Below there is an introduction to a number of examples of these three types of modern herbal drinks, and, later, some recipes to help you try making some of your own.

Examples of Modern Herbal Drinks

Absinthe

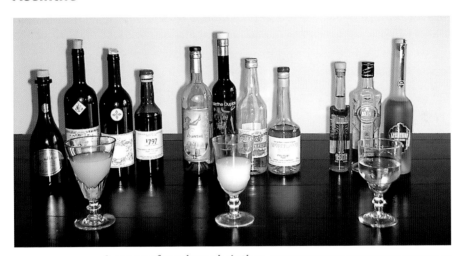

A range of modern absinthes. BRIAN ROBINSON, WORMWOOD SOCIETY, CC

With its vibrant green colour, absinthe is instantly identifiable. It conjures up romantic images of Paris at the turn of the century, when it was enjoyed by many of the great artists and writers of the era. Originally from Switzerland, it was initially sold as a medicinal spirit and, much like gin, it was used as a malarial preventive. By the 1880s, mass-production techniques made it both cheap and widely available, and its medical origins were largely forgotten as it became closely associated with hedonistic overconsumption.

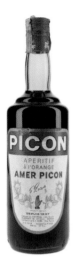

Amer Picon

This drink was originally created in 1837 by Gaétan Picon, a Cavalry sergeant in the French army. After falling ill in Algeria with malarial symptoms he reportedly treated himself with a herbal tea of orange peel, sugar and quinine. Impressed at the success of his concoction, he took the same ingredients and mixed them with alcohol, which was then widely drunk by French soldiers across North Africa to fight malaria. He went on to open a distillery later in life in Marseilles where he produced Amer Picon for sale to the general population.

Amer Picon, a French aperitif flavoured with bitter orange and gentian root.

Amaro

Amaro is a popular Italian digestif with a bitter-sweet flavour. There are a range of types available in supermarkets, each of which uses a slightly different blend of roots, herbs and fruits. The ingredients are first macerated in alcohol before being matured in oak barrels to add flavour. These recipes have evolved from similar drinks that were produced in monasteries across Europe and sold in apothecaries. For Amaro recipes to try at home, *see* later in this section.

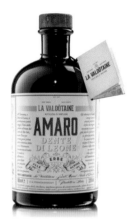

Amaro from a small distillery in the Aosta Valley, Italy.

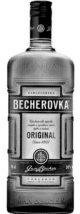

Becherovka

Becherovka is a popular herbal bitter that is enjoyed as a digestif. It was created in the Czech Republic by Josef Becher, who was a trader in herbs and a physician, and later in life became a distiller. The recipe was and remains a closely guarded secret, with only one or two people knowing the full process and ingredients used in its production. Although there are apparently more than twenty herbs and spices used in the recipe, the predominant notes that come through are cinnamon and ginger – anyone who feels up to the challenge could try to produce their own version! It was originally produced to help alleviate the symptoms of stomach diseases but is now enjoyed predominantly for its taste. A popular way to serve it is with tonic water and ice, much like gin.

Becherovka.

Benedictine

Developed in France by Alexandre Le Grand, Benedictine was marketed as being based on herbal recipes from a local monastery and uses over twenty-seven types of flowers, berries, roots and herbs. Interestingly, the English town of Burnley in Lancashire is one of the most lucrative markets for this liqueur, where it is enjoyed with hot water and known as 'Bene 'n' Hot' or 'Benny and Hot'. This is the result of a large number of soldiers from Burnley being stationed in the First World War near the Benedictine Abbey at Fécamp in Normandy, where the spirit is said to have been developed.

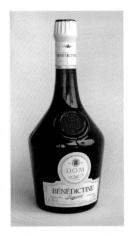

Benedictine, a herbal liqueur made to a recipe that came from a monastery in the sixteenth century. It contains a blend of 27 herbs and spices.

CHRIUSHA/WIKIMEDIA COMMONS

Buckfast Tonic Wine

Buckfast is a well-known caffeinated fortified wine that is infamous across the UK, particularly in Scotland, where it has unfortunately become associated with heavy drinking and anti-social behaviour. It was originally produced by Benedictine monks at Buckfast Abbey in Devon, who were influenced by recipes brought over from France by other monks of the same order. In the 1920s production shifted from the monastery to a local wine merchant, where it was sold in small quantities and marketed as a health product under the slogan, 'Three small glasses a day for good health and lively blood.'

Chartreuse

This French herbal liqueur is available in green and yellow variations. It has been made by Carthusian monks since 1737 to a secret recipe that uses 130 herbs and spices. That recipe dates back to 1605 and is said to be derived from an ancient concoction that was used as a medicinal drink and reputed to lead to longevity. It is named after the Grande Chartreuse monastery, which is located near Grenoble in France, in the Chartreuse Mountains. The monks still make a

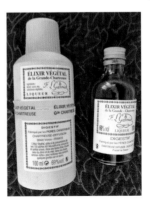

Chartreuse Elixir Medical, a concentrated herbal drink made by Carthusian monks containing 130 herbs and spices.

ZEPHYRIS/WIKIMEDIA COMMONS

much stronger digestif *elixir medical*, which is used in much smaller quantities for medicinal purposes.

Cynar

This is a well-known Italian herbal aperitif that can be found behind most Italian bars. Developed by the Campari group in the 1950s, it is made from a blend of herbs and could be considered a type of Amaro. The liquor is based on the leaves of the globe artichoke, whose Latin name *Cynara scholymus* gives it its name. Recent research into the artichoke has led to the discovery of the bitter-tasting compound cynarin, which has been found to stimulate digestive secretions, making it very suitable as an aperitif drink.

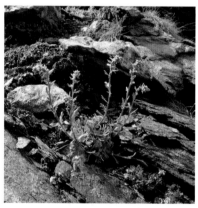

Alpine wormwood, the vital ingredient of genepi.

Genepi

Traditionally, this is a drink that is made from steeping herbs in alcohol, which is then sweetened and drunk as a digestif. Originating in the Savoy region and the Aosta Valley, its distinctive flavour comes from the inclusion of alpine species of *Artemisia*, or wormwood. It was traditionally made by local families, and many of the recipes remain a closely guarded secret to this day.

Hierbas

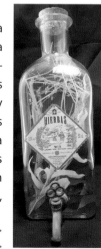

Hierbas means 'herbs' in Spanish, but the term also refers to a range of herbal drinks that originate from northern Catalonia and the Balearic Islands. They were initially created for therapeutic purposes by monks and, whilst certain key ingredients are always included, the exact recipes differ from monastery to monastery and place to place. Often, locally available herbs and berries are used. Hierbas are sweetened and drunk as a digestif in small amounts. Key to their distinctive flavour is green anise, which has a unique flavour that is the result of high concentrations of essential oils such as anethole and estragole,

Hierbas: with the herbs left in to be preserved by the alcohol. It is a very bitter herbal tonic made to an ancient recipe.

all of which have been shown to reduce flatulence and nausea. Hierbas will also frequently contain peppermint, another strong-tasting herb with a calming effect on the digestive system.

Jägermeister

Jägermeister is perhaps one of the best-known herbal spirits in both the US and the UK. It has been successfully marketed to become a favourite of young drinkers in clubs and pubs across the globe. It is actually another drink that comes from the tradition of using alcohol to preserve therapeutic plants. Developed just over eighty-five years ago in Germany by a vinegar company, it contains a mixture of fifty-six different herbs, which give it its signature flavour. Although, like many of these drinks, its exact recipe remains a closely guarded secret, it is known to contain herbs that aid the digestive system, such as star anise and cinnamon. It is unusual amongst herbal spirits in being aged in oak barrels, not unlike whisky, which gives it a strong woody flavour.

Izarra

Izarra is a sweet liqueur originating from Bayonne in the French Basque country. The recipe was developed by French botanist Joseph Grattau in the late nineteenth century from local recipes that date back much earlier. Grattau started to produce it commercially at the beginning of the twentieth century, naming it Izarra (which means 'star' in the Basque language). Izarra is a barrel-aged distilled infusion of Pyrenean herbs and macerated walnut shells and prunes in Armagnac. This once local drink is now commercially produced by a large international drinks company.

Patxaran

Patxaran is a Basque liqueur, from the Spanish part of the region. It is a digestif that began life as a popular local drink made by macerating sloes, cinnamon and coffee beans in anisette (a liqueur flavoured with aniseed and other locally sourced herbs). It was known to be drunk in Navarre as early as the Middle Ages and its ongoing popularity is thought to stem from home-made varieties being taken by young men doing their national service.

Swedish Bitters

Unlike many of the commercialized brands, Swedish bitters, sometimes known as Swedish tonic, is one alcoholic drink that is still valued for its therapeutic benefits. The recipe, which combines large numbers of familiar herbs such as angelica root and saffron, also contains unusual ingredients such as Venetian theriac. This

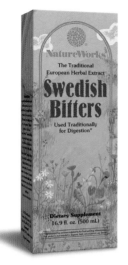

is an ancient mixture of herbs that was traded across Europe and Asia as a 'cure-all'. Created in Sweden in the eighteenth century, Swedish bitters was claimed to be based on a remedy by an ancient Greek physician named Paracelsus. It remained associated with health rather than recreation largely due to the efforts of Maria Traben, a well-known herbalist, who wrote a number of best-selling books in the 1980s. She deserves much of the credit for the increased interest in herbal remedies across Europe at that time.

Swedish bitters.

Underberg

Underberg is a German sweetened digestif, first produced in 1846. It has enjoyed continuous popularity in the country, with production being interrupted only by the Second World War. Unfortunately, this is another drink whose exact recipe is kept as a closely guarded secret but, like Jägermeister, it is known to be matured in oak barrels. Unusually, it is still classified under oils, herbs and spices rather than as an alcoholic drink, meaning that it can be sold without an alcohol licence and so is widely available across Germany to this day. Typically, it is sold in small 20cl bottles and is traditionally used to promote a healthy digestive system.

Unicum

Unicum is a popular Hungarian herbal liqueur and is considered to be one of the country's national drinks. Made in Budapest using a blend of forty herbs and spices, it is oak-aged for six months, giving it a similar flavour to both Underberg and Jägermeister. The recipe is attributed to the Royal Physician of the Austro-Hungarian imperial court, Dr József Zwack, who created it in 1790 as a therapeutic beverage for the health of the digestive system. It received the royal seal of approval and went into commercial production in 1840, after which, due no doubt to the association with the imperial court, it quickly became a popular product.

Vermouths

Vermouths are fortified wines that contain a blend of herbs and spices. There are two main forms: a red sweetened version and an unsweetened white dry version. There are many commercially available brands of vermouth that are drunk as aperitifs or used as ingredients in several popular cocktails, including negronis and martinis. They were originally produced in apothecaries as medicinal drinks in and around Turin in the eighteenth century, where they were made by steeping a range of herbs in fortified wine. The name derives from the French pronunciation of the German *wermut*, or wormwood, which is the central ingredient in vermouth, providing both its distinctive flavour and its therapeutic effects. Hippocrates, the father of modern medicine, recommended worm-wood for the treatment of intestinal parasites.

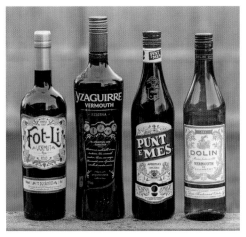

A range of vermouths.
KENNETH C. ZIRKEL

Recipes

Amaro Recipes

There are three different amaro recipes below and you are encouraged to play around and create some of your own. These recipes are designed to make relatively small amounts for your own consumption. It is important to note that, if you are planning to produce larger amounts for commercial sale, you will need to pay much closer attention to the concentration of alcohol in your finished product.

You will need the following equipment:

- a large cooking pan (big enough to contain 2 litres of water);
- a large sealable container (either a glass demijohn or a food-grade plastic bucket with lid);
- muslin cloth;
- sieve;
- large measuring jug;
- clean glass bottles with lids;
- funnel;
- kitchen scales.

Ingredients

For Fresh Summery Amaro:

5g dried orange peel

1 star anise

5g cinchona bark

5g dried cherries

2g fresh sage leaves

2g fresh basil leaves

3g grains of paradise

The zest of two fresh oranges and two fresh lemons

100g sugar

2 litres 40% alcohol (cheap vodka is best, as it has a relatively neutral flavour)

50g toasted oakwood chips

For Spicy Amaro:

5g dried orange peel

6 cardamom pods

3 cloves

12 juniper berries

3g dried gentian root

5g white pine bark

3g dried mint

5g dried cranberries

2g fresh ginger

1 small cinnamon stick

100g muscovado sugar

2 litres 40% alcohol (cheap vodka is best as it has a relatively neutral flavour)

For Herby Amaro:

5g dried orange peel

1 star anise

4 cardamom pods

3g dried angelica root

2g wormwood

2g dried hyssop

2g dried artichoke leaf

1 fresh sprig lemongrass

The zest of one orange, one grapefruit and one lemon

6 fresh mint leaves

100g sugar

2 litres 40% alcohol (cheap vodka is best, as it has a relatively neutral flavour)

Method

1. Bring 2 litres of water to the boil in the large pan. Lower the temperature to keep it simmering and add the sugar, stirring until it has completely dissolved. Cover with a clean cloth and leave to cool to room temperature.
2. Weigh out all the ingredients and combine with the sugar and water mixture in a large sealable container.
3. Add 2 litres of 40% alcohol to the mixture and seal the container. Leave for at least three weeks in a cool, dark place.
4. When it is ready, the mixture needs to be strained into a large measuring jug, using a sieve and some muslin cloth.

5. Once the mixture has been strained, you can begin bottling up. Carefully clean the bottles you are planning to use, to prevent contamination, and use a funnel as it can get messy.
6. When sealed, the bottles will keep for at least a year.

Vermouth Recipes

As with amaro, the process of making your own vermouth is surprisingly simple and yet can be incredibly rewarding. Vermouth is made up of fortified white wine that has been flavoured with fruit and herbs and spices. You then have the option of adding a sugar and water mixture to create sweet vermouth, or leaving out the sugar to create a dry vermouth.

This vermouth recipe is designed for home use. If you want to produce it commercially, the ABV (alcohol by volume) will need to be calculated, as with the elixir recipes (*see* Chapter 5). It is usually made at between 15% and 20% ABV. This recipe uses a blend of herbs and spices that we have enjoyed, but feel free to add any that you think will add a distinctive flavour to your own version.

You will need the following equipment:

- a large pan with a lid;
- an old pan to use to caramelize the sugar;
- a large sealable container (either a glass demijohn or a food-grade plastic bucket with lid);
- sieve;
- muslin cloth;
- a large measuring jug;
- clean glass bottles with lids;
- funnel;
- kitchen scales.

Ingredients

(To make approximately 2 x 70cl bottles)

1.5 litres dry white wine (you can use cheap wine as you are going to flavour it, but make sure it is not oaked)

0.4 litres of dry sherry

The zest of two large oranges, one lemon and one grapefruit

7 cardamom pods

2 cloves

2 sprigs of fresh thyme

1 star anise

1 cinnamon stick

3g fresh wormwood

1 sprig of fresh rosemary

2g dried sweet orange peel

150g sugar

Method

1. Measure out 0.5 litres of white wine and gently warm it in a large pan.
2. Carefully weigh out all the herbs and spices and add to the pan of wine. Gently simmer for 15 minutes.
3. Take the pan off the heat and allow to cool to room temperature.
4. In the old pan, mix the sugar with a small amount of water on a medium heat. Keep stirring until it caramelizes, turning into a thick brown syrup.

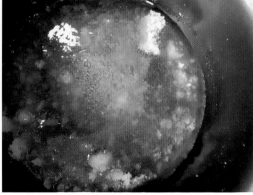

Caramelized sugar.

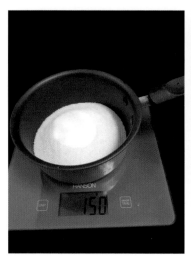

Weighing out sugar.

5. Leave this mixture to cool and then add 200ml boiling water and stir well to dissolve the caramel.
6. Using a sieve lined with muslin, strain the herbs and spices from the pan of wine into a large measuring jug.
7. Add the caramelized sugar and water mixture, the sherry, and any leftover wine to the mixture, stir well.
8. Fill sterilized bottles, using a funnel.

Part 2

Techniques

3

Picking and Storing Herbs

Herbal elixirs are blends of syrups and tinctures that have been chosen for their medicinal properties and flavour. Of course, there are many tinctures and syrups available to buy, but the process of growing or foraging your own herbs and preserving them yourself can be an enjoyable and rewarding experience. This chapter will explore how and when to pick herbs and how to preserve them by making tinctures or syrups. Syrups are made by dissolving sugar in boiling water, and herbs and fruit can then be preserved in this solution. Tinctures use an alcohol solution to extract and preserve the active elements in herbs and roots.

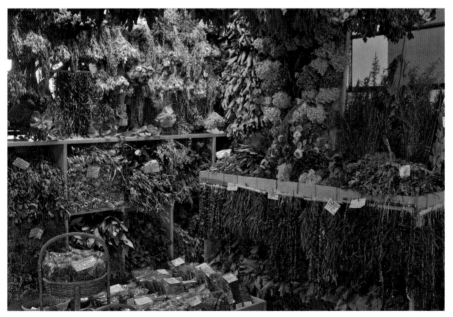

Dried herbs in a market. Drying is the easiest way to preserve them.

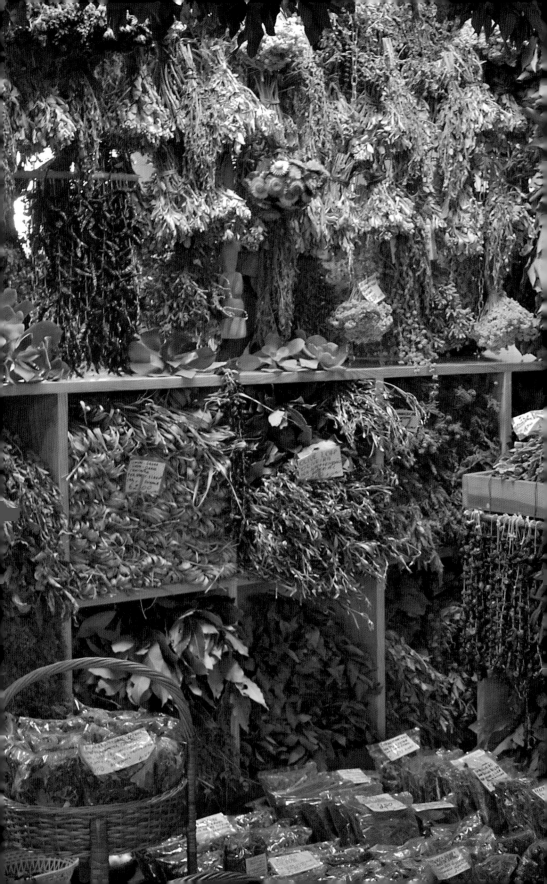

Harvesting and processing herbs correctly and efficiently is a crucial part of making potent plant extracts to use in herbal elixirs. Whether using dried or fresh plant material, the most important thing is to ensure that it is organic, biodynamic or grown wild. If wild picking, ensure the plants are a good distance away from main roads and fields that have been sprayed with chemicals. Pesticides and herbicides are organic chemical compounds and they will be extracted and concentrated when the plant material is steeped in alcohol. These compounds are used to kill pests and weeds and they also have a negative effect on human health. Many have been linked to the development of certain diseases, including cancers.

Where possible, it is preferable to use freshly picked plant material in your tinctures and syrups. This leads to a fresher, more vibrant flavour and means you are extracting the compounds at their most effective. In most cases, however, dried or frozen plants are easier to access. As long as they are from a reputable supplier, they will still produce a good result. Luckily, there is an abundance of reputable companies supplying a wide variety of herbs from across the world (*see* Appendix II for a list). They provide a great way to get hold of herbs that are out of season, hard to find growing wild, or rarely cultivated in the UK.

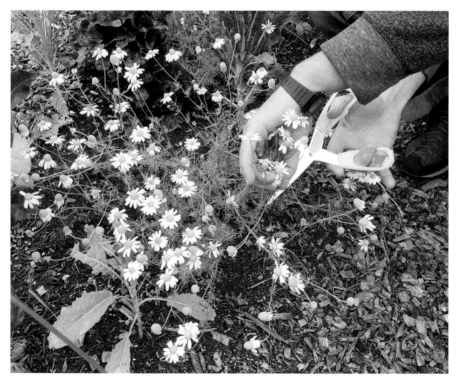

Picking fresh chamomile flowers for drying.

Selecting and Picking Herbs

The elixir recipes are inspired by myriad ancient remedies. For each unique blend, inspiration has been drawn from traditional British herbal medicine, as well as from Chinese medicine and the Indian Ayurvedic medicine, to create balanced drinks with herbs that complement each other therapeutically and that taste great when combined. When selecting the herbs and plants to use in your elixirs, it is best think about the flavour of the drink as well as the traditional medicinal benefits. If you are not sure which herbs to combine, have a look at the chapter on herbal monographs as a guide. You can also book a consultation with a qualified herbalist for advice on tinctures tailored to your personal requirements. It is most important that your elixir should taste good as well as making you feel good.

There are certain parts of a plant that are best harvested at a particular time of year. This can be because this part is available only during a short period, or because it contains more active compounds than the rest of the plant in a certain season. The recipes given here will specify where necessary which part of the plant to use. For some herbs, such as echinacea, it is the roots that contain the active ingredients. In others, it is the seeds (for example, in fennel), or the leaves (in mint), the flowers (lime) or even the fruit (schisandra). To decide which part of the plant to harvest and when, refer to the herbal monographs at the end of the book or consult a qualified medical herbalist.

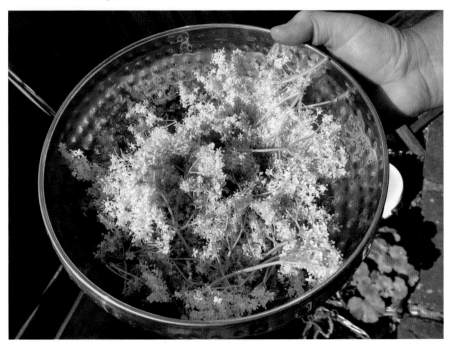

Flowers of the elder, picked to make elderflower syrup.

The aerial and flowering plants are usually harvested in summer when the sun is at its height. The roots of annual and biennial plants are best harvested in the autumn, when they are at their most robust, as they store energy for the winter. There are exceptions, however; perennial plants are best harvested in the spring before the plant begins growing its stem. If you are growing these yourself and can track their growth, it is recommended that they are left until their second year of growth, so the root is fully developed.

Preserving and Storing Herbs

There are many ways of preserving delicate leaves and flowers. Whichever method you decide to use, start by gently washing the plant matter, or simply shake off any bugs and dirt.

Leaves and Flowers

Freezing

Freezing plant material is a very effective way of preserving it. Do it as soon as possible after harvesting as this will greatly improve the qualities and capture some of the vibrancy of the flavour and scent of a freshly picked herb. When freezing delicate leaves or flowers, use a rigid, sealable container like a Tupperware to prevent bruising or breakages. For more robust plant matter, such as roots, fruits or berries, a bag should suffice. After defrosting, use the material as soon as possible as it will quickly begin to lose its flavour.

Syrup

Whether in the form of granulated sugar, honey or glycerine, sugar is an excellent preservative. Syrups make use of this quality and are made by dissolving sugar in boiling water. Herbs and plants can then be added and cooked in this solution. Stored correctly – in sterilized jars in a cool, dark space – they will last for up to a year. For further information on this process, *see* Chapter 5.

Tincture

Alcohol is an excellent preservative and provides the most efficient and longest-lasting way to keep plant material. Tinctures are a combination of dried or fresh herbs each with a specific ratio of water and pure grain alcohol. When making tinctures, it is vital to pay careful attention to the ratio of water to alcohol as it varies from plant to plant. *See* the table in Chapter 5 for more information on this.

Infusing

Infusing herbs into water is essentially the same process as making herbal tea. It works best with more delicate leaves, berries and flowers. Simply add one cup of water for every teaspoon of herbs, bring to the boil and simmer for 10 to 15 minutes. This can be stored in the fridge for up to two days but it should be discarded if you notice any change in the liquid. These are more immediate herbal remedies and will not store well for long as they have no preservative element.

Decocting

A decoction is essentially the result of infusing hard, woody roots and herbs in water to make something similar to a really strong cup of tea. Dried herbs will need to be decocted for longer and you can use less than you would for fresh herbs, as the fresh version contains more water and is less concentrated. When a recipe calls for one part of dried herb, if using fresh herbs use three parts instead.

Start by adding the dried or fresh plant material to water in a saucepan, at a rate of one teaspoon for every cup of water. Bring to the boil and simmer for 10 to 20 minutes. This will give you a potent infusion. You can also cold- or solar-infuse a decoction. Add dried or fresh plants to water and put in the window for up to 12 hours. The heat of the sun will help to extract the flavour and the water-soluble constituents.

Dehydrating

A great way to preserve fresh leaves and roots is to dry or dehydrate them. You can do this in a number of ways, for example, by spreading thinly on a tray on a sunny window or by hanging a full bunch of flowers upside down in the window until they have dried. Alternatively, you can use a dehydrator. The more resourceful can make their own by following one of the many tutorials to be found online.

Once the material is dry, store it in an airtight container away from direct sunlight and use it to create a tincture or a syrup. Use it within a year for the best results.

Roots

When harvesting the roots of a plant, take care to clean them carefully before use. You can simply wash them under a tap or in a bowl of water, but if you are processing a large amount you can bundle them up into a muslin cloth or a clean cotton pillowcase and put into the washing machine. Select a short cycle, cold wash, with no soap, and they will come out clean and ready to use.

Once clean, they can be used fresh or they can be frozen, dried or turned into a syrup or tincture, in the same way as leaves and flowers.

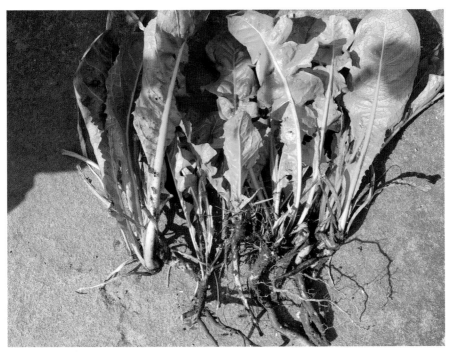

Dandelion roots before cleaning.

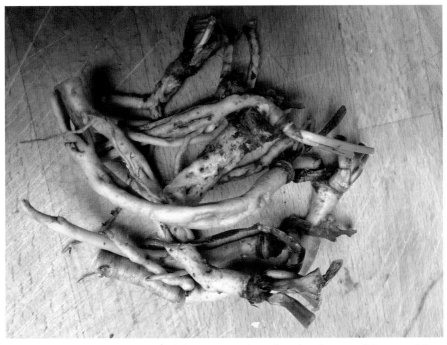

Dandelion roots after cleaning in a washing machine.

Fruits

When it comes to selecting fruit, choose organic and pick them at the peak of their growth, in order to preserve them during times of their seasonal abundance. Wash the fruits and freeze or turn into a syrup (*see* above). Both are excellent ways to store fruits until you are ready to make your elixirs.

Seeds

When harvesting the seeds from plants, you can use them fresh, or employ the same methods as described above to dry and dehydrate them to use at a later date.

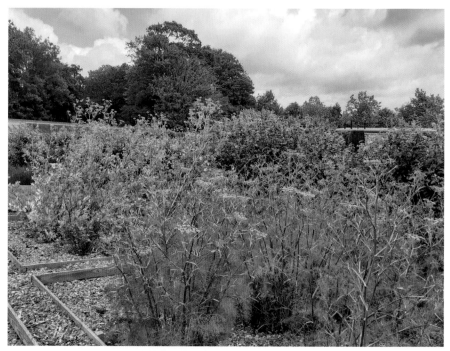

Fennel plants with seeds ripe and ready to pick.

Foraging in the UK

Below is a month-by-month guide to some plants that are commonly found growing across the UK and are suitable to be harvested and used in herbal remedies and drinks. Foraging provides the perfect additional activity to any trip to the countryside, whether it is a cycle ride or a dog walk. Once you know what to look for, you will find that you are always stumbling upon useful and delicious plants.

An increasing disconnection from the environment has caused the knowledge and practice of foraging to be largely forgotten and that lack of knowledge often brings with it anxiety. There are a few basic points to bear in mind when you are out that will help keep both you and your environment flourishing.

Always take care not to pick or consume a plant unless you are completely sure that you have correctly identified it. You can limit the chances of this by taking a comprehensive local botanical guide with you, by engaging with the many vibrant online communities on social media platforms such as Facebook, or by joining local foraging walks. You should also make sure that you are harvesting the correct part of the plant. There can be a big difference in the chemical make-up of the different components of certain plants.

Make sure that you take into account the area where you are foraging. For example, avoid picking too close to busy roads as the fumes can accumulate in the plants, potentially causing health issues. Harvesting plants that are close to sites of industrial agriculture can also bring its own set of issues, as the herbicides and pesticides that are used will often spread to plants nearby. These chemicals can be harmful when consumed and they will be extracted and concentrated by the processes used to preserve plants. Finally, for obvious reasons, you may want to avoid low-lying plants in areas that are popular with dog walkers.

To promote the health of the plants you are harvesting and to allow others to enjoy them as well, you should look to forage in areas that have an abundance of the plants that interest you, and then only take enough for your personal use. When possible, try to limit the damage by not stripping individual plants, instead taking a small amount from a number of plants. Be mindful, too, not to disturb wildlife or damage their habitats.

For a more complete guide to plants and herbs that can be foraged, take a look at the herbal monographs in Chapter 7.

January

With its short days and cold weather, January can often be a gloomy time of year in the UK, and it is easy to think that foraging might be a rather fruitless activity during this month. However, while it is true that many plants and herbs grow seasonally and will therefore be unavailable, the resourceful forager will always find something. In fact, this is the perfect time of year for harvesting the barks of certain trees and hedges.

As it is often difficult to identify trees in winter, when they are without their leaves or fruit, it is a useful tip to spot and note the relevant examples in your area in the other seasons. In the summer, this can be done by looking at their foliage, and in the autumn the berries will be a good indicator.

The two trees described below grow commonly across northern Europe and their bark has a number of well-documented therapeutic uses. To harvest the bark, you will need a sharp knife. Peel it off in small vertical strips and do not take too much from one area, as this could leave the tree open to harmful fungal infection.

White Willow (*Salix alba*)

White willow is a large, deciduous, fast-growing tree generally found along a watercourse. In summer, it can easily be identified by its distinctive pale green leaves. The use of willow bark as an analgesic and anti-inflammatory has a long history and it has also been found to be effective in the treatment of a variety of fevers. You can either dry it and add it to teas or soak it in alcohol to create a tincture.

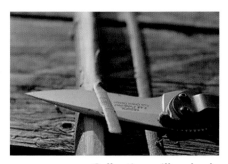

Collecting willow bark.

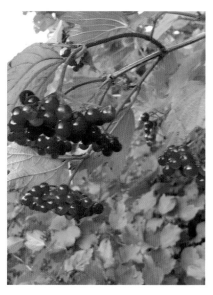

Guelder Rose (*Viburnum opulus*)

Also known as 'cramp bark', this is a large deciduous bush or small multi stemmed tree that is commonly found in hedgerows in the south of the UK. In summer it can be identified by its white, pom-pom-like flowers, and in the autumn it has bright red berries. As the common name suggests, its bark has been used for most types of muscular tension; it has proved particularly useful in the treatment of menstrual cramps.

The bright red berries of *Viburnum opulus* in the autumn.

February

By February, plants in the UK are slowly starting to come to life. As the days get longer, this can be the perfect time to think about collecting roots. Choose a day without frost and pack a small trowel when you go out. You will often find that, thanks to the UK's notoriously wet winters, the ground will have been softened by rain, making plants easy to lift.

When you are removing the roots, take extra care not to harvest all the plants in one area, as they may well not grow back. This will damage the local environment, as well as preventing other foragers from being able to harvest their own supply.

Dandelion (*Taraxacum officinale***)**
Although it is often treated as a weed and thrown straight on to the compost heap, all parts of the humble dandelion – flowers, leaves, stems and roots – are actually very useful. Dandelion leaves are rich in potassium and have traditionally been used as a diuretic. They can also be enjoyed as part of a salad or cooked and added to meals. The vibrant

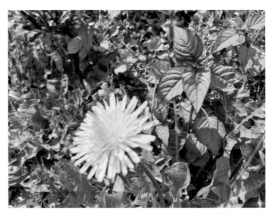

Dandelion (*Taraxacun officinale*).

yellow flowers of the plant can also enhance a dish, for example, when they are fried and added to an omelette. Even the roots can be used. Perhaps most popular is to use the root to make a cordial but they can also be roasted and ground into a caffeine-free coffee substitute. Tinctures made from the roots are used to treat liver complaints.

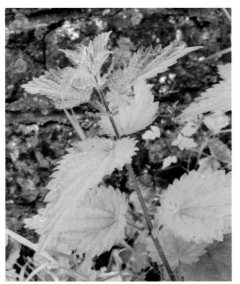

Nettles (*Urtica dioica***)**
Known best for their irritating sting, nettles are another versatile favourite of the forager. At this time of the year, before the leaves have fully grown, you can still harvest the roots for making tinctures. Research has indicated that nettle roots can be effective in the treatment of urological disorders.

Nettles (*Urtica diocea*).

March

With spring well on its way, the month of March is accompanied by lengthening days and a sudden burst of greenery across the woodland floor as it drinks in the light that is allowed in through the still-sparse leaves of the trees above. This is the perfect time of year to collect the many leafy herbs that grow in and around hedgerows and to seek out the herbs and plants of the woodlands.

Nettles (*Urtica dioica*)

Choose the young nettles, which are packed full of iron and many other minerals and vitamins. Use gloves to avoid getting stung, and remember to pick in clean areas, away from roads, agricultural activity and dog walkers. The leaves are best enjoyed in a delicious iron-rich nettle soup. They are considered to help reduce inflammation and pain around the joints and were traditionally beaten against joints to treat arthritis.

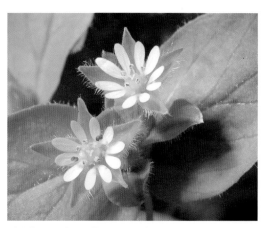

Chickweed (Stellaria media).

Chickweed (*Stellaria*)

Chickweed is a familiar garden weed recognizable by its tiny white flowers. The seeds were once fed to birds, which is how the plant earned its common name. A great way to make use of this abundant weed is to harvest the leaves and the delicate white flowers. They are full of vitamins and minerals and make a good addition to an early spring salad. Medicinally, chickweed is used as an anti-inflammatory. A tincture made from the leaves and flowers is often added to a base to make a very effective skin cream. It is soothing for eczema, sunburn and insect bites as well as being useful in drawing out splinters and boils.

Cleavers (*Galium aparine*)

Commonly known as 'sticky weed', cleavers have a tendency to 'cleave' to human clothing or animal fur. The young, bitter leaves and stems can both be harvested. The plant is rich in vitamin C and was used as a vegetable when other greens were still not ready to sprout. It can be used to create a tincture that will have a powerful astringent and diuretic effects.

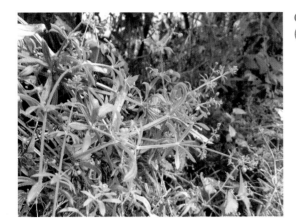

Cleavers, or goose grass (*Galium aparine*).

Gorse (*Ulex europaeus*)

These vibrant yellow flowers have a distinct coconut smell and taste. They can be used to add a wonderful aroma and flavour to an elixir. The beautiful yellow flowers can be found growing wild on sunny, sandy clifftops and heathland.

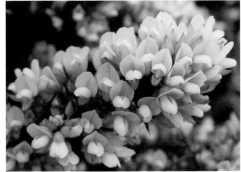

Gorse flowers (*Ulex europea*).

April

As the days continue to lengthen and warm, the possibilities for foraging grow almost as quickly as the plants. By April, there is widespread flowering and a wealth of culinary herbs begin to bloom. In particular, this time is marked by the distinctive aroma of wild garlic as it fills UK woodlands. Wild garlic does have health benefits and can be used to make delicious soups and pestos, but it is too strong to include in any elixirs, where its flavour would be overwhelming. Fortunately, there are many other herbs that can be foraged in April.

Marshmallow (*Althea officinalis*)

If you mostly associate marshmallow with the sweet treat that is used to top hot chocolate or toasted over an open fire, you might be surprised to learn that its parent plant is a very useful one in herbal medicine. As the name suggests, it is found in waterlogged areas such as bogs and marshes. Although it does not flower until later in the summer, the leaves and roots can be harvested in spring. They all contain large amounts of mucilaginous compounds, which can be used to

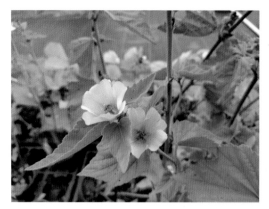

soothe inflammatory conditions of the gut. Marshmallow is rich in calcium, iron and vitamin C and has traditionally been used to soothe bad coughs and sore throats.

Marshmallow (*Althea officinalis*).

Peppermint (*Mentha piperita*)

Peppermint is a hybrid of water mint that is grown in many gardens. Water mint (*Mentha aquatica*) is a very common plant found in wet ground. The leaves are best harvested at this time of year before the plants flower. Peppermint relaxes the gut and can help relieve indigestion and nausea.

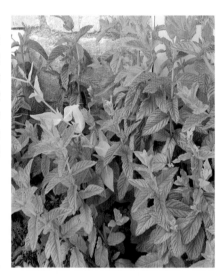

Mint (*Mentha piperita*).

May

May is a beautiful month right across northern Europe. The formerly forlorn, skeletal branches of the deciduous trees are suddenly laden with vibrant leaves and blossoms. There is no time of the year when the countryside looks greener than during this first burst of colour. After a long winter, the scent of the blossoms and early budding flowers means that the trees are a delight to the nose as well as the eye. May is the month when you can catch some of the short-lived blossoms of trees such as the linden, which will make a fantastic addition to any herbal concoctions that you might feel inspired to create.

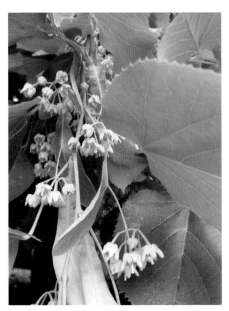

Lime flowers (*Tilia europea*).

Lime (*Tilia europaea*)

Commonly called linden trees, these are not to be confused with the lime trees that produce the citrus fruits. They are actually large, beautiful deciduous trees that are often found in English parkland. Their flowers are fragrant and can be eaten raw, or they can be used to add a fragrant, citrus flavour to an elixir. They are said to have a sedative and calming effect on nerves and muscles and can reduce tension and anxiety. The flowers will appear only for a few days so you must be quick to harvest them, although they can be frozen to preserve their freshness until you are ready to use them.

Red Clover (*Trifolium pratense*)

Red clover can be found growing abundantly in parks and open grassland. It is the red, sweet-smelling and sweet-tasting flower heads that are harvested. Red clover has traditionally been used for women's hormonal ailments as well as treating skin conditions, due to its purifying effects. The flowers are known to contain oestrogenic steroids and can be used to alleviate some of the discomfort caused by the menopause.

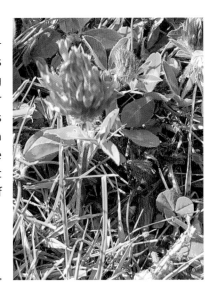

Red clover (*Trifolium pratense*).

Elderflower (*Sambucus nigra*)

These sweet-scented flowers can be found growing abundantly in parks, woodlands and hedgerows right across the UK. Elderflowers are particularly well suited to making a fresh and fragrant syrup and are a common ingredient in home-made

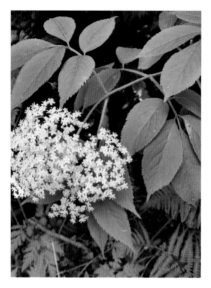

cordials. They will add a burst of fragrant sweetness to an elixir that will make it irresistible. In herbal medicine, the flowers are used to reduce mucus production, helping to relieve the symptoms of hayfever, a common complaint at this time of year.

Elderflower (*Sambucus nigra*).

June and July

With summer well and truly here, these are the months to venture outdoors in earnest. Why not combine camping, walking or a little wild swimming with some foraging? There is perhaps no better medicine than a beautiful summer's day spent outside enjoying the beauty of the countryside with friends or family, stocking up on some good memories to sustain you through the winter months. For foragers, this is a particularly abundant time of year, with many plants and herbs ready to harvested. It is a good idea to take a small container or a cloth bag with you wherever you go, as you never know when you might stumble across something useful!

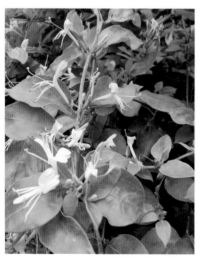

Honeysuckle (*Lonicera periclymenum*)

The beautiful fragrant flowers of honeysuckle are best used to create a delicious syrup to sweeten your elixirs. Honeysuckle can be found growing in hedgerows and is recognizable by its distinctive tubular flowers. Take care to harvest the flowers only as the berries are mildly toxic and are best avoided. Honeysuckle has traditionally been used to treat chest ailments and is used for a wide variety of problems in Chinese medicine.

Honeysuckle (*Lonicera periclymenum*).

St John's Wort (*Hypericum perforatum*)

St John's wort is a small deciduous plant that is native to the edge of woodlands and hedgerows in Europe. The flowers produce a red juice when crushed, giving the plant its name, as the juice is said to be associated with the blood of St John the Baptist. It can be a little tricky to identify, but a good distinguishing feature is a perforated appearance to the leaves when they are held up to the light, caused by a proliferation of tiny oil glands. It is often used externally for various skin conditions as a tincture but is perhaps best known as a treatment for mild depression. In particularly, it is widely used to treat the symptoms of SAD (seasonal affective disorder), a common complaint in the northern hemisphere.

Plantain/Ribwort (*Plantago lanceolate*)

This is a very common plant and gardeners spend a lot of time pulling it up and putting it on the compost heap, as it is a very invasive weed. However, it can be a useful herb. The leaves have been used medicinally since the Middle Ages, as they contain mucilaginous compounds that can soothe both the digestive system and the respiratory system.

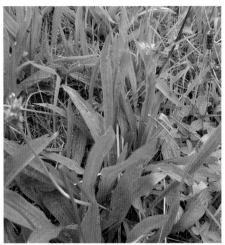

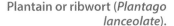

Plantain or ribwort (*Plantago lanceolate*).

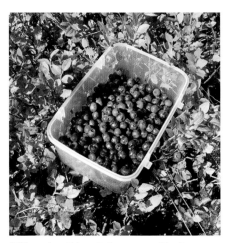

Bilberries (*Vaccinium myrtillus*).

Bilberries (*Vaccinium myrtillus*)

Usually found in mountainous or hilly areas, these delicious and very sweet berries may be small, but they pack a powerful punch. They can be made into either a tincture or a syrup, although a syrup will best preserve the flavour. They have an extremely high vitamin B, C and A content, are considered to contribute to fine blood vessel health and are rich in antioxidants. They have also been used as a laxative when fresh, so it is important to take care not to overindulge!

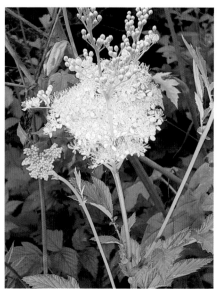

Meadowsweet (*Filipendula ulmaria***)**
The beautiful almond-scented creamy white flowers of meadowsweet are found growing abundantly along road verges, hedgerows and canal towpaths. It was from these flowers that salicin was first isolated in 1838 by Felix Hoffman. His employer, Bayer, named this drug 'aspirin' after the old botanical name for meadowsweet – *Spiraea ulmaria*. Tinctures made from meadowsweet are useful for the treatment of fevers and to alleviate muscle and joint pain.

Meadowsweet (*Filipendula ulmaria*).

August

As the year moves later into the summer, there are more berries and fruits on the trees and bushes. Again, it can be a good tip to take a container with you to collect any berries that you might find on walks and cycle rides. This can be a very rewarding time to forage, as berries are easy to pick, so even young children can join in.

Rowan or Mountain Ash
(*Sorbus aucuparia*)

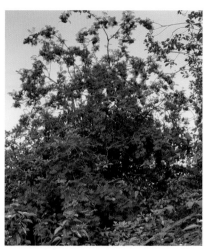

The bitter red-orange berries of the rowan grow in clusters on trees in woodland and parks. They can be used to make a drink with a very interesting flavour, but they must be turned into a syrup beforehand, as they are inedible when raw. Take particular care to remove all of the seeds prior to using the berries, as they are toxic.

Rowan tree with berries (*Sorbus aucuparia*).

Damson or Bullace (*Prunus domestica*)

Damson and bullace trees were originally domesticated but can now often be found in hedgerows. Bullaces are a round shape and smaller than the oval damsons. Their main characteristic is a distinctive rich flavour. In common with all purplish fruits, they are rich in antioxidants but, unlike plums, they are both high in sugars and highly astringent. They can make a tasty and sweet addition to your elixirs.

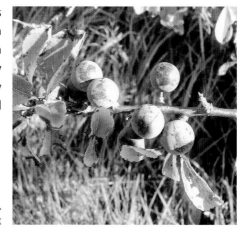

Ripe damsons (*Prunus domestica*).
EVELYN SIMAK

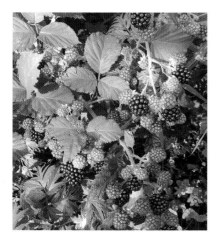

Blackberries (*Rubus fructicosa*)
Blackberries grow wild in great abundance in hedgerows across England. They are beautifully sweet and will add a rich tart note to an elixir. As a bonus, they are powerful antioxidants and packed full of a wide array of vitamins and nutrients.

Blackberries/brambles (*Rubus sp.*).

Hawthorn (*Crataegus* **spp.**)
Hawthorn is popular as a quick-growing hedge plant. The bright red berries are one of the oldest medicinal plant ingredients that are known to be packed full of antioxidants. As they are inedible raw, they must be turned into a sweet syrup or tincture before use. Tinctures made from the berries are used by herbalists to treat various problems such as cardiac weakness, hypertension and heart palpitations.

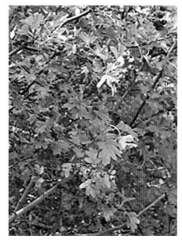

Hawthorn berries (*Crataegus sp.*).

September

Marking the end of summer and the beginning of autumn, September can be a beautiful month in the UK. The shifting colours of the foliage and crisp, clear autumnal mornings and evenings make it one of the forager's favourite months. It is a fantastic time for foraging, as the last flowering of the summer provides many berries, seeds and fruits. It is, after all, Keats's 'season of mists and mellow fruitfulness'.

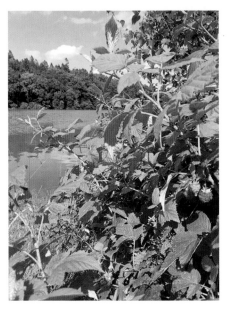

Wild Raspberries (*Rubus idaeus*)

Growing abundantly in woodlands and hedgerows right across the country, raspberries are easily identified. If you manage to get any home without eating them all beforehand, make a fantastically tasty syrup. You can also use the leaves to make a tincture. Raspberries are full of vitamins and antioxidants.

Wild raspberries (*Rubus idaeus*).

Elderberries (*Sambucus nigra*)

Found in woodlands around the UK, and particularly prevalent on the towpaths that run alongside the many miles of canals that criss-cross the English countryside, the elder tree produces deep purple berries. They are best prepared in much the same way as the flowers early in the year – turned into a syrup, which will add a depth of flavour and sweetness to an elixir.

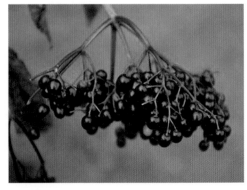

Elderberries (*Sambucus nigra*).

Care must be taken to cook them thoroughly, as they are inedible raw. Elderberry syrup has been used throughout history to relieve symptoms of cold and flu.

Hops (*Humulus lupulus*)

Wild hop vines may be found in hedgerows across southern Britain, particularly in the county of Kent in the south-east of England. It is the fruiting bodies that ripen in the late summer and early autumn. They have been bred to produce different species that are grown in hop gardens and used to add flavour in the brewing of beer. Known for bitter and citrussy notes, they have

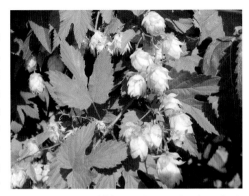

Wild hops (*Humulus lupulus*).
DR HAGEN GRAEBNER

been used in remedies to promote restful sleep and relaxation. Take care to use only small amounts of the tincture when making mixtures as the flavour is quite powerful and can overwhelm others.

October

With the nights really starting to draw in, this is the last month when foraging can still be a rewarding exercise, so it is important to make the most of it! Like September, it is a time for berries and seeds, with a few late blooming flowers in the mix. It can be beneficial to health and well-being to maintain a connection with the outdoors at this time of year, and resist the urge simply to batten down the hatches and stay at home. The conditions outdoors usually look worse from the inside than they really are, so wrap up warm, dig out a pair of wellies, put on your raincoat and go out and see what you can find!

Maidenhair (*Ginkgo biloba*)

The maidenhair is a hardy deciduous tree that was introduced into Europe early in the eighteenth century. It grows well in Britain and is frequently found in parkland and in many gardens. Its fan-shaped leaves turn a beautiful bright yellow in the autumn. Extensive research has identified many pharmacological effects of ginkgo leaves, which are best collected in the autumn after they have changed colour. The tincture made

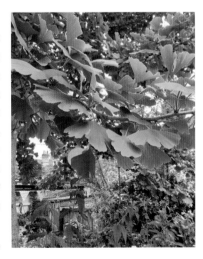

Ginkgo tree (*Ginkgo biloba*).

from the leaves is used for a range of conditions, from poor concentration and memory problems in older people to the symptoms of respiratory illnesses such as asthma.

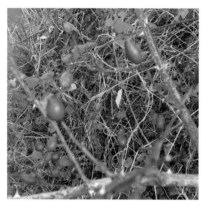

Rosehips (*Rosa canina*)

The bright red fruits of the wild dog rose can be seen in hedgerows across Britain. In fact, once you know what you are looking for, you will undoubtedly start to see them everywhere! It was once very common to use rosehips to make a syrup for children to be taken throughout the winter months, as they are rich in vitamin C and are delicious.

Rosehips (Rosa canina).

Blackthorn (Sloes) (*Prunus spinose*)

If you look in any hedgerow you will most likely find a blackthorn bush. Its fruits are small purple plum-like sloes. They make an amazing syrup, although the bush's long thorns can make harvesting a hazardous business. The sweetness of the syrup helps to bring out the flavour of the sloes and they create an elixir that has a beautiful colour. Traditionally, it is thought best to pick the fruit after the first frost.

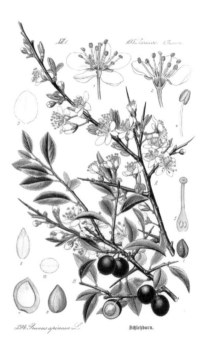

Botanical illustration of sloe flowers, fruit and seed by Otto Thome, 1885.

November and December

In these winter months, most plants are dormant and foraging is an unrewarding activity.

4

The Manufacture of Alcohol

Fermentation and Distillation

'Alcohol' is often used as a blanket term for drinks that have an alcoholic content, and you could be forgiven for thinking that there is only one type of alcohol. In fact, there are many different forms. It is very important to bear this in mind as some – for example, isopropyls – are highly toxic and should *not* be consumed under any circumstances. Mostly, when the term 'alcohol' is used, it actually refers to ethanol. Ethanol has been produced and consumed by humans for thousands of years. It is safe to consume in small amounts and makes up the alcoholic content of beers, wines and spirits. It has a number of properties that make it a fantastically useful substance and it is an essential part of

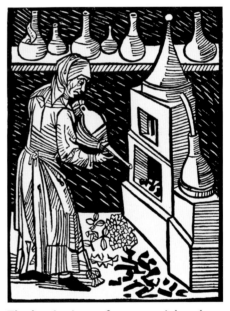

The beginnings of commercial-scale alcohol distillation.

creating herbal elixirs. While alcohol is probably best known today for producing a headache the morning after the night before, its properties as both a solvent and preservative make it a vital tool in the hands of any aspiring herbalist. This dual ability is ethanol's time-saving superpower, allowing the simultaneous *extraction* and *preservation* of the active elements of herbs.

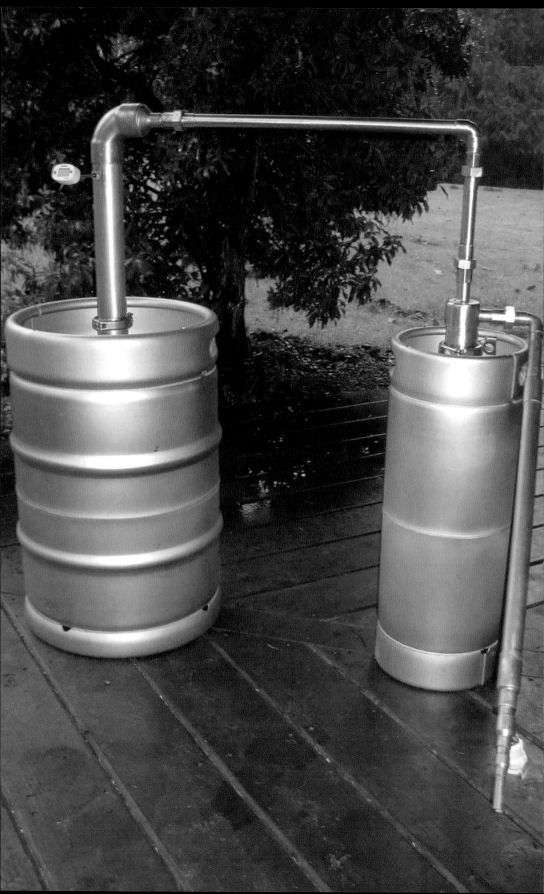

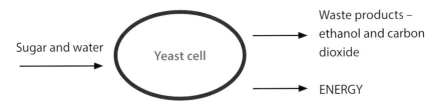

Sugar and water → Yeast cell → Waste products – ethanol and carbon dioxide

→ ENERGY

The fermentation process within a yeast cell.

It is possible to produce ethanol through certain types of fermentation. The term 'fermentation' may conjure up the image of bubbling vats in wineries or breweries, but in reality it is a chemical process that is happening all around us, all the time, and even *inside* of us. Fermentation stands alongside photosynthesis and aerobic respiration as a chemical process that allows energy stored in molecules to be released; all three are absolutely essential to life on earth.

There are broadly speaking two types of fermentation: the type that is harnessed in the brewing industry to produce alcohol, and the type that produces lactic acid, which is experienced as a burning sensation in the muscles during intensive exercise. The herbalist needs to focus only on the first type!

Using fermentation to produce alcoholic drinks has been a mainstay of human activity across the world for thousands of years. All sorts of raw materials, from mare's milk in Mongolia to cacti in Mexico, have been fermented, but it is only relatively recently that the actual process and organisms behind it have been discovered and understood. Aristotle, in many ways the founder of the structure of modern scientific enquiry, was reportedly fascinated with fermentation, concluding that it was a distinct life force at work. However, it was French chemist and microbiologist Louis Pasteur who discovered the microscopic organisms busily at work producing alcohol: this was the living yeast that transformed glucose into ethanol. This discovery allowed far greater control over the fermentation process and, eventually, the selective breeding of specialized yeasts that are suited to different tasks.

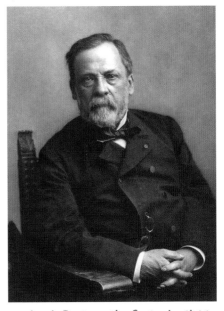

Louis Pasteur, the first scientist to understand that alcoholic drinks are the result of yeast transforming glucose into ethanol.

However, fermentation alone is not able to provide the strength of alcohol that is needed to make herbal elixirs. There is a natural limiting factor (and irony) in that, while the hard-working yeast creates alcohol simply by virtue of being alive (fermentation is yeast's 'breathing'), it cannot survive in solutions above a certain alcohol percentage. It is the endless and regrettable fate of the yeast organisms to drown in their own excretions. This means that it is not possible to produce alcoholic concentrations of higher than around 12–14% through fermentation alone, before the yeast dies and thus stops fermenting. Fortunately, this problem has been solved by the ingeniously simple concept (but often complicated task!) of distillation.

Distillation is a technique that separates different components of a solution by exploiting different boiling points. By heating the solution up to the boiling point of the desired product, it is possible to alter its state from liquid to gas. If this gas is then captured and cooled, the result will be a liquid containing a far higher concentration of the desired product than the initial solution. The effect of the liquid passing through the apparatus gave the process its name, from the Latin verb *destillare*, meaning 'to drip' or 'trickle down'.

Much like fermentation, distillation is a process that has been used in various different forms across the world for thousands of years. Although the process has always been more or less the same, the methods and apparatus used have varied significantly, from a simple open vessel heated over a fire with a cloth or sheep's wool held over the top to catch the vapour, which is then squeezed out into a separate vessel, to a complicated set-up involving a network of pipes and tubes. The most enduring type of apparatus – the alembic still – is believed to date back to the tenth century, when it was developed by Arabic alchemists and later spread across Europe. So successful is this design that it is still frequently seen in use today, in an almost unchanged form.

Producing and Distilling Your Own Alcohol

The process of producing and distilling alcohol can be divided into two parts. First, you need to create a solution that can be fermented in order to produce the alcohol. This solution is called a mash. It consists of ingredients that have a high sugar or carbohydrate content – for example, fruit, grains or vegetables – which are mixed with water and the all-important yeast. This stage is very important in the production of many spirits, such as whisky, as the ingredients chosen and the conditions in which they are fermented all impart a particular flavour and quality to the end product.

Second, you have to distil the fermented mash to arrive at your final product. This a relatively simple process in theory, but it can be complex in practice, as there are many ways to approach the task, all of which will produce different flavours and qualities of spirit. However, as your aim as a herbalist is to produce alcohol that will be infused with herbs, you need to create a simple spirit without any special flavours. As a result, the process should remain relatively simple: choose a still, make a mash and distil a final product!

Step 1: Choosing a Still

The complete range of stills available and the different sums of money that you could pour into them would make for a long list. However, if you are simply looking to produce small amounts at home for personal use, there are some very affordable options out there.

Basically, there are three different types that are suitable for smaller quantities: air stills, bucket or 'moonshine' stills, and alembic stills. There are also commercial stills, which have a greater capacity (*see* below).

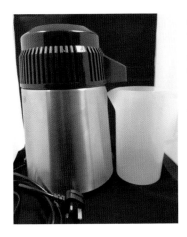

Air Still

The air still suits those looking to make smaller quantities of alcohol on a relatively low budget. They can be picked up for around £150–200. With an internal heat source and temperature control, this type of still is by far the easiest to use.

An air still – the simplest and cheapest still that can be purchased.

Bucket or 'Moonshine' Still

Based around home-made stills used by resourceful booze hounds during prohibition in America, the bucket or 'moonshine' still is simple, cheap and hard-wearing. However, unlike the air still, it does require both an external heat sources and cold-water supply. It also lacks an automatic thermostat to control

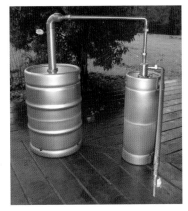

Moonshine still – there are a variety of moonshine still designs. They are generally produced in the USA.

the temperature; instead, the heat is controlled by adjusting the settings on the kitchen hob whilst keeping a beady eye on the thermostat. This means that a bucket still is both more complicated to set up and involves far more attention during distilling.

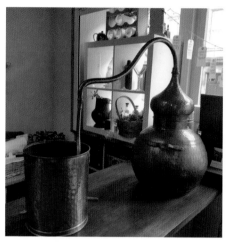

Copper alembic still – the most traditional design of still.

Copper Alembic Stills

Alembic stills can be bought in a range of sizes, from as little as one litre to as large as 50 litres. They are significantly more expensive than the other two options described above, but they are beautiful objects in their own right, as well as being durable and sufficiently hard-wearing to last the careful user a lifetime. Like a bucket still, an alembic still requires both an external heat source and a cold-water supply, and the temperature will have to be controlled by adjusting the kitchen hob in accordance with the temperature readings on a thermometer.

Commercial Stills

Commercial stills have a much larger capacity and are far easier to control, allowing a consistently high-quality product to be reliably reproduced. They can be fully automated, with a complex system of sensors monitoring temperature, alcohol strength, and testing for impurities in the distillate. They can vary in size from 150 litres, for use in smaller craft distilleries, to more than a thousand litres. These huge stills are used in large industrial distilleries of well-known brands.

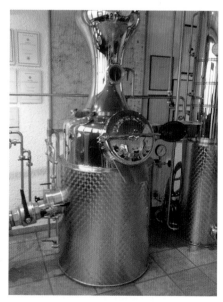

A 125-litre modern commercial pot still made in Germany by Kothe.

Step 2: Making the Mash

Anything with a high sugar or carbohydrate content can be used to create a mash, although it is worth bearing in mind that some mashes will require the addition of enzymes to help break down more complex sugars for the yeast to feast on. If you do decide to use different ingredients and methods from those shown below, it is worth researching your mash thoroughly to avoid the disappointment of a failed fermentation. The mash described below will not need the addition of any enzymes, as sugar is added directly into the solution. This is often referred to as a 'sugar wash'. The method below will produce around 20 litres of mash, as this is usually the quantity that a standard individual packet of yeast is designed to make.

Choosing your Yeast

It is worth bearing in mind that, if you want to achieve the best results, you cannot just use any old yeast. Even the briefest of internet searches will tell you that there are a bewildering number of yeasts sold by home brewing sites. There are, however, two that are most highly recommended: a turbo yeast, like the Classic 8, which is a best-selling yeast all over the world, and is capable of producing an alcohol yield of up to 18%; and the widely available distiller's gin yeast, designed for creating craft spirits such as rum, gin or vodka. The latter will also produce a clean neutral spirit that will be perfect for showcasing the flavours of your chosen infusions.

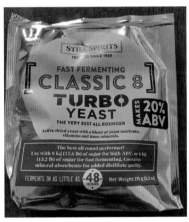

A packet of turbo yeast.

For the best results, it is vital to read and follow carefully any instructions that come with the yeast, as different types will have different optimum conditions for fermentation. The method shown below uses distiller's gin yeast, as this is often the easiest to find in shops and online.

Equipment

You will need the following equipment for fermenting a mash:

- fermentation bucket;
- thermometer;
- short length of flexible tubing;
- kitchen scales;
- large measuring jug.

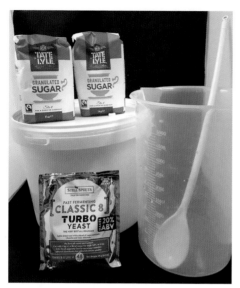

The equipment required for making a mash.

The mash can sometimes be fermented within the central container of an air still or a bucket still. However, for many stills you will need a separate container or fermentation bucket. There are a number of suitable products that can be bought from home brewing shops or online, but a food-grade plastic tub of an appropriate size with an airlock is recommended. The airlock will allow carbon dioxide produced through the fermentation to escape, whilst at the same time stopping oxygen from entering the tub. You will also need a short length of flexible tube that can be used to siphon the finished mash into your still for distillation.

Ingredients

1 sachet of turbo yeast
6kg granulated sugar
Clearing agent (optional)

21 litres water
Small bag of ice cubes

Method

Before starting, thoroughly clean out the container or fermentation bucket with boiling water and soap, to ensure that there are no lingering bacteria, which might derail your fermentation.

Combine the sugar and water in the fermentation bucket. To ensure that the sugar is fully dissolved, heat or boil the water just before adding the sugar and stir vigorously. This creates the sugar wash.

Before adding the yeast, make sure that the temperature of your sugar solution is between 20 and 32 degrees centigrade. This is very important, as adding the yeast when the temperature is too high will kill many of the yeast cells and prevent a successful fermentation. To lower the temperature, either wait for the solution to cool down on its own, or add ice cubes slowly to the mix until the temperature is within the desired range.

Once the mix is at the correct temperature, add the yeast. Again, stir it well until it dissolves into the sugar wash.

Once the yeast is thoroughly mixed in, place the lid of the fermentation bucket on firmly, taking care to check that it has seated properly. Leave the mixture to ferment for approximately seven days, taking care that the temperature stays at between 20 and 32 degrees centigrade. You will know when fermentation has stopped as the mixture will stop bubbling.

Finally, let the sediment in the wash settle. You can do this either by leaving it to stand for one to two days or by using a clearing agent, which will speed up the process. Clearing agents are available from home brewing shops both online and on the high street.

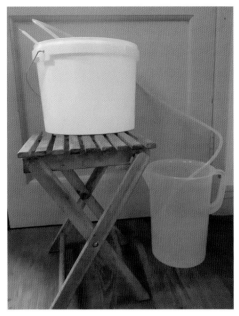

Syphoning off the mash to leave the yeast residue behind.

Once the sediment has settled, the sugar wash is ready to be carefully siphoned off for distilling. Take care not to disturb the sediment as this can affect the next step.

Step 3: Distillation

Once you have created the sugar wash, the next step is to run it through your still. As the distillation process will vary according to the type of still that you have chosen, it is very important to read or watch the appropriate instructional material before firing up your still and starting your first distillation. It is not possible here to explore thoroughly all the methods relating to all the different types of still that exist, but it will be useful to focus on the general principles of distillation. These remain the same, no matter what kind of still is used.

Not all the distillate produced is usable or desirable. In fact, the process and its products are divided into four different stages: the foreshots, the heads, the hearts and the tails. The skill of the distiller lies in being able to determine at which point these stages begin and end, and in making a 'cut' at those points. With each 'cut', the distiller will replace the container collecting the distillate, making sure that there is no cross-contamination between them. This is a skill that takes practice, and requires a mixture of observation and judgement – this is why distillation is often described as 'part science, part artistry'.

Below is a detailed description that will help you make your own 'cuts' and set you on your way to becoming an accomplished distiller!

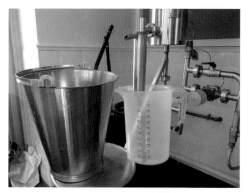

Measuring the heads and foreshots before collecting the hearts of the still run in the bucket.

Foreshots

The very first vapours to be collected, even before the heads, are called the foreshots. Great care should be taken to ensure that they are never included in your final collection as they contain methanol, a type of alcohol that is harmful when consumed. The foreshots make up around 5% of the final still run and can be identified by their strong solvent smell.

Heads

Next come the heads, which will generally make up roughly 20% of the liquid collected during distillation. Like the foreshots, they contain undesirable alcohols such as acetone, which, although they are not as harmful as methanol, will contribute to a head-splitting hangover if consumed. The heads can be identified by a strong solvent-like smell and an oily texture when rubbed between the fingers. Like the foreshots, you will want to take care not to include these in your final product. Whilst the percentage guides can give a good indication of the amounts of heads to expect, the best way to make the right cut is to check the product frequently by smell and feel. Always err on the side of caution, as it is best to lose a little of the hearts in the heads than it is to allow the heads to lower the quality of your final product.

Hearts

This is the stage of the distillation that produces the desired product – ethanol. The hearts should make up around 40% of the distillate, and can be identified by the change in smell as the solvent-like aroma of the acetone is replaced by the sweeter smell of ethanol. This is a game of the senses. A skilful distiller is able to maximize the amount of hearts captured by quickly identifying these shifts in smell, texture and taste.

Tails

The last 30–35% of a still run is known as the tails. Again, you will need to use your senses to recognize the changes in the products you are capturing. The shift from hearts to tails is accompanied by an oily film that collects on the surface of the distillate and a burnt, smoky smell and taste. The tails contain proteins and carbohydrates from your wash that you do not want in your final product.

Whichever type of still you have used, the hearts that you will have collected from your run will be between 75 and 95% ABV. This product needs to be stored in a suitably sized glass or food-grade plastic container with a good seal, as the alcohol evaporates easily and is highly volatile. It must be kept in a safe place, away from any sources of open flame, as it is very flammable.

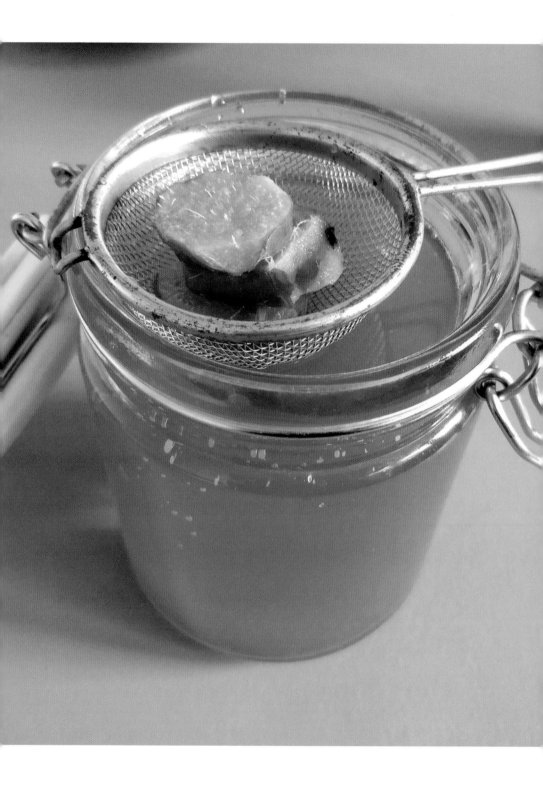

Part 3

Recipes

5

Making Tinctures and Creating Syrups

Making Tinctures

Background

Making a tincture is a way of extracting the chemical compounds found in herbs that form the basis of medicinal treatment within the Western tradition of herbal medicine. A tincture is typically an extract of a root, leaf, flower or seed of a plant, extracted in alcohol using concentrations of 25–60% ABV.

To make a tincture, the plant parts are left to steep in a mixture of alcohol and water. The percentage of alcohol to be used depends upon the chemicals to be extracted from the herbs. In order to make your elixirs you will need to make tinctures of individual herbs that you can then blend together and sweeten. Plants are very complex chemical entities, whose composition is studied in the science of phytochemistry. The

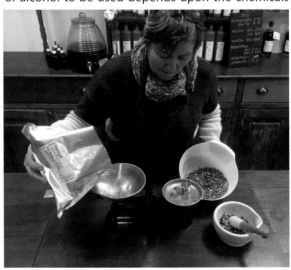

Weighing out dried herbs to make tinctures.

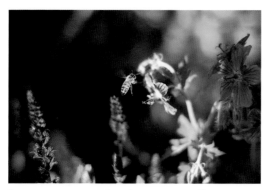

Bees are attracted to flowers to collect nectar and pollen.

aim in making a tincture is to extract the useful medicinal compounds – generally the secondary plant metabolites. These are chemicals that plants produce in order to attract insects, to facilitate seed dispersal, or to act as a defence against microbial or fungal attack.

For many years, scientists in the pharmaceutical industry have extracted and extensively researched these plant metabolites. Some chemicals can be synthesized and form the basis for a large proportion of the pharmaceutical products available today. This research continues, with plant-derived drugs being developed all the time. During the last decade, new drugs on the market have exploited such products as arteether, a semi-synthetic natural derivate of artemisia (wormwood), which has been effectively used in malarial treatment. Galantamine, a natural alkaloid obtained from *Galanthus nivalis* (the snowdrop), is being used in the early treatment of Alzheimer's disease. Apomorphine is a semi-synthetic compound derived from morphine (itself derived from *Papaver somniferum*, the opium poppy), which has had some success in the treatment of Parkinson's disease. Tiotropium, a derivative of atropine from *Atropa belladonna* (deadly nightshade), is now commonly prescribed for chronic obstructive pulmonary disease. Capsaicin, the active compound from *Capsicum annuum* (cayenne pepper), is manufactured and marketed as an analgesic for pain relief.

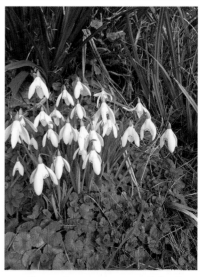

Snowdrops are one of the first signs that winter is drawing to a close and spring is on the way.

The most striking feature of natural products in connection to their long-lasting importance in drug discovery is their structural diversity, which is still largely untapped. When a tincture is created, the beneficial chemicals are extracted in a form that can then be used to make a herbal elixir. Unlike the pharmaceutical industry, which aims to isolate individual chemicals that can then be synthesized and produced commercially, the herbalist is using whole plants and extracting all of their chemical constituents. Herbalists believe that the various constituents often work together and that the medicinal benefits are the result of a synergistic interaction of all of the chemicals. In herbal medicine, this interaction is felt to be more powerful than any individual component acting alone.

Sourcing and Selecting Plant Material

Wild Harvesting
When sourcing fresh herbs, it is very important to pick them only from somewhere you know to be free from chemicals. Be aware that herbs growing close to a road can be affected by the particulate pollution that many vehicles produce. Correct plant identification is essential as plants that look alike can have very different chemical constituents. Some plants, even within the same family, may look very similar but have vastly different properties. For example, it is quite difficult to distinguish wild carrots from hemlock – and the latter is a deadly poison. There are many books available with excellent keys that can help make identification easier, using botanical features such as leaf shape, colour and flower structure. It is also important to know and use the Latin names, as common names can often vary from region to region.

Growing Your Own
Growing your own is probably the most satisfying way to source your herbs. Many of the herbs that can be used in elixirs are relatively easy to cultivate. After harvesting, they can be dried and stored for future use. Harvesting is the fun bit of growing your own herbs – roots in the autumn and green tops as they start to emerge, flowers in the summer and seeds once they are ripe, but before they start to disperse, and fruits when they are as ripe as possible but before they start to drop or rot.

Buying Dried Herbs
A dried herb of good quality should always be organically sourced, as both herbicides and pesticides are organic chemicals that are very easily taken into solution by alcohol. As a result, they are prone to being concentrated in tinctures. Check that any leaves or flowers are as close to the original colour as possible. They will start to fade with age, and this will make them less effective. There should be recognizable plant parts and not too much dust. Powdered herbs are often all that are available, but the process used to produce them generally shortens the shelf life.

Practical Method for Making a Tincture

Making a tincture is a straightforward process but there are a couple of important things to bear in mind when you are preparing the ingredients. When using fresh herbs, take care to wash them carefully to remove any soil or insects. Roots can be placed in a pillowcase and put through the washing machine on a short, cold wash, with no cleaning products added. They should then be finely chopped or they could be made into a paste with a stick blender.

If you are using dried herbs, you can grind them into smaller pieces in a pestle and mortar. This increases the surface area and, in turn, the amount of the chemicals that can be taken into solution.

Equipment

Large kilner jars or food-grade plastic bucket
Dried or fresh herbs (organic)
Measuring cylinders
Measuring jug
Pestle and mortar
Scales
Alcohol of known strength
Distilled water
Calculator
Muslin squares
Funnel
Bottles with swing tops
Labels

Method

Use the table below, showing the alcoholic strengths of common tinctures, to decide on the ABV of the tincture you are going to make.

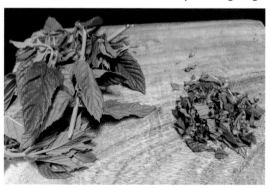

Grind the dried herbs to a fine powder in a pestle and mortar. If using fresh herbs, cut up finely.

Weigh the fresh or dried herbs and place into either a suitably sized kilner jar or a food-grade plastic bucket.

Cutting up fresh herbs.

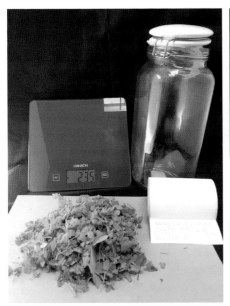

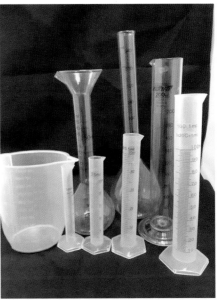

The cut herbs are weighed and then added to an accurately labelled and sterilized jar.

A range of accurate measuring cylinders and jugs.

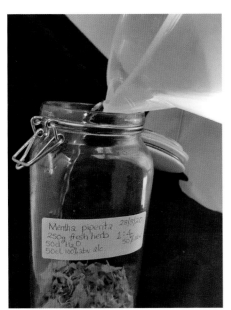

Measured amounts of alcohol and distilled water are added and carefully recorded.

Combine a carefully measured amount of alcohol at a known ABV to distilled water to arrive at the strength recommended in the table below. (For advice on the process for altering the strength of an alcohol solution, *see* the end of the chapter.)

Carefully label the jars or buckets and store in a dark place.

After three to four weeks, empty the jars and strain the contents through muslin cloth into a clean measuring jug. Bottle the finished tincture into clean glass bottles, preferably of a dark colour, to prevent sunlight from degrading the chemicals and reducing the effectiveness of the tincture.

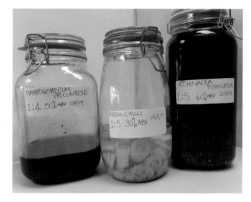

The labelled jars can be placed in a dark storage space.

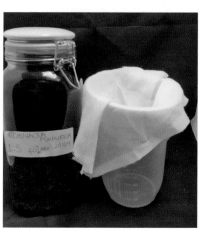

Place a muslin square in a sieve to strain the macerated herbs, to create the tincture.

Alcohol Strengths

Recommended Alcohol Strengths for Common Herbs

Various alcohol strengths are used when making tinctures of the common herbs. The percentage ABV means the ratio of alcohol to water in the solution to be used.

Herb	% ABV	Herb	% ABV
Althea officinalis	25%	Hypericum perforatum	45%
Apium graveolens	60%	Matricaria recutita	40%
Astragalus membrosa	25%	Mentha piperita	45%
Capsicum species	45%	Panax ginseng	45%
Carduus marianus	25%	Rheumania glutinosa	25%
Cimicifuga racemosa	25%	Salix alba	25%
Cinamomum zeylancia	45%	Salvia officinalis	45%
Echinacea purpurea	25%	Schisandra chinensis	25%
Foeniculum officinalis	40%	Withania somnifera	25%
Ginkgo biloba	25%	Vaccinium myrtillus	25%
Glycyrrhiza glabra	25%	Verbena officinalis	45%
Harpogophytum procumbens	40%		

Calculating Alcohol Strengths

To make a tincture using a solution of alcohol at different strengths (ABV), you will need to carry out some calculations. The ABV for a tincture is determined by the chemicals in a particular herb that need to be drawn out into solution. The alcohol mixture is usually either 25% or 45% ABV – with a few exceptions – so you may need to alter the strength of the alcohol that you have either made or bought.

Before you can bring your alcohol mixture to the required strength, you will need to know its current strength. If you are working with store-bought alcohol, this is simple, as all commercially sold alcohol has its ABV clearly labelled. However, if you are working with home-distilled alcohol, you will need to use a piece of equipment called a hydrometer. This is a calibrated glass tube with a bulb on the bottom, used to measure the density of a liquid solution, enabling you to calculate the strength of an alcoholic mixture. The more alcohol there is in a mixture, the less dense it is, so that the hydrometer will sink lower. The less alcohol in the mixture, the more dense it will be, and the higher the hydrometer will sit in the solution. Hydrometers are carefully calibrated to indicate the exact percentage of alcohol to water in a solution.

Hydrometers vary greatly in terms of both price and accuracy. You can buy a cheap one from any home brewing shop, which will give you an approximate ABV that will be sufficient for home production. If you are going to produce elixirs commercially, your ABV measures need to be very accurate and you will require an expensive hydrometer, a thermometer and a set of alcohol tables.

The method for using a hydrometer and calculating the ABV from the reading is as follows:

1. Put a small amount of the alcohol mixture into a sample jar and take its temperature.

2. Carefully place the hydrometer in the jar, letting it float. Wait until it is no longer moving, then read off the scale to find the ABV. When reading a hydrometer, you should look at where the meniscus of the liquid shows against the scale on the hydrometer, and take the reading from the lowest point (*see* illustration).

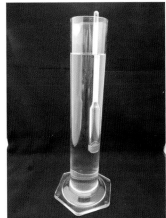

A hydrometer in a measuring jar filled with alcohol.

3. When you have both the temperature and the hydrometer reading, use the alcohol tables (*see* opposite) to work out the ABV.

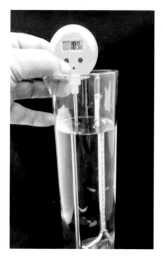

A digital thermometer will give the most accurate temperature reading.

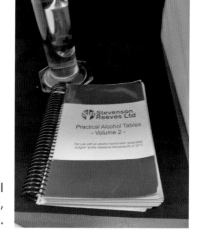

Alcohol tables are used to calculate alcohol percentages (*Practical Alcohol Tables*, Volume 2, Steveson Reeves Ltd).

The alcohol tables are laid out with a set of temperatures running across the top and hydrometer readings in the vertical column. Using your temperature and hydrometer readings, you can find the strength of your alcohol. For example, if the temperature is 18.9 degrees centigrade and the hydrometer reading is 948.8, tracing down from the temperature and along from the hydrometer indicates that the strength of the alcohol solution is 43.5% ABV.

Making Your Alcohol Solution

Once you know the ABV of the alcohol that you are going to use to make your tincture, you can use the following formula to calculate how much distilled water you will need to add to make an alcohol solution of the correct strength (ABV).

It is worth noting that it is best to use distilled water, as it is free from all contamination, both chemical and biological. You can buy distilled water (which is often used to fill car batteries), distil it yourself or, on a bigger scale, use a reverse osmosis filtration system.

Using the alcohol tables to get an accurate measurement of the ABV.

ρ* \ t	17.5	18.0	18.5	19.0	19.5	20.0
			IX b q = q (ρ*,t)			303
940.0	45.7	45.5	45.3	45.1	44.9	44.7
940.2	45.6	45.4	45.2	45.0	44.8	44.6
940.4	45.5	45.3	45.1	44.9	44.7	44.5
940.6	45.4	45.2	45.0	44.8	44.6	44.4
940.8	45.3	45.1	44.9	44.7	44.5	44.3
941.0	45.2	45.0	44.8	44.6	44.4	44.2
941.2	45.0	44.8	44.7	44.5	44.3	44.1
941.4	44.9	44.7	44.5	44.3	44.1	44.0
941.6	44.8	44.6	44.4	44.2	44.0	43.8
941.8	44.7	44.5	44.3	44.1	43.9	43.7
942.0	44.6	44.4	44.2	44.0	43.8	43.6
942.2	44.5	44.3	44.1	43.9	43.7	43.5
942.4	44.4	44.2	44.0	43.8	43.6	43.4
942.6	44.2	44.0	43.9	43.7	43.5	43.3
942.8	44.1	43.9	43.7	43.5	43.3	43.1
943.0	44.0	43.8	43.6	43.4	43.2	43.0
943.2	43.9	43.7	43.5	43.3	43.1	42.9
943.4	43.8	43.6	43.4	43.2	43.0	42.8
943.6	43.7	43.5	43.3	43.1	42.9	42.7
943.8	43.5	43.4	43.2	43.0	42.8	42.6
944.0	43.4	43.2	43.0	42.8	42.6	42.4
944.2	43.3	43.1	42.9	42.7	42.5	42.3
944.4	43.2	43.0	42.8	42.6	42.4	42.2
944.6	43.1	42.9	42.7	42.5	42.3	42.1
944.8	43.0	42.8	42.6	42.4	42.2	42.0
945.0	42.8	42.6	42.4	42.3	42.1	41.9
945.2	42.7	42.5	42.3	42.1	41.9	41.7
945.4	42.6	42.4	42.2	42.0	41.8	41.6
945.6	42.5	42.3	42.1	41.9	41.7	41.5
945.8	42.4	42.2	42.0	41.8	41.6	41.4
946.0	42.2	42.0	41.8	41.7	41.5	41.3
946.2	42.1	41.9	41.7	41.5	41.3	41.1
946.4	42.0	41.8	41.6	41.4	41.2	41.0
946.6	41.9	41.7	41.5	41.3	41.1	40.9
946.8	41.8	41.6	41.4	41.2	41.0	40.8
947.0	41.6	41.4	41.2	41.0	40.8	40.6
947.2	41.5	41.3	41.1	40.9	40.7	40.5
947.4	41.4	41.2	41.0	40.8	40.6	40.4
947.6	41.3	41.1	40.9	40.7	40.5	40.3
947.8	41.2	41.0	40.8	40.6	40.4	40.2
948.0	41.0	40.8	40.6	40.4	40.2	40.0
948.2	40.9	40.7	40.5	40.3	40.1	39.9
948.4	40.8	40.6	40.4	40.2	40.0	39.8
948.6	40.7	40.5	40.3	40.1	39.9	39.7
948.8	40.5	40.3	40.1	39.9	39.7	39.5
949.0	40.4	40.2	40.0	39.8	39.6	39.4
949.2	40.3	40.1	39.9	39.7	39.5	39.3

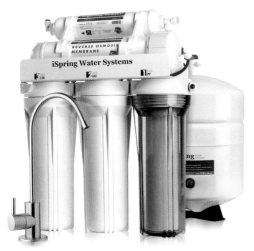

Reverse osmosis equipment to produce distilled water.

The formula to work out how much distilled water to add is as follows:

Starting volume of alcohol in litres x (current ABV ÷ final ABV required) = Total volume (litres)

Total volume – starting volume = amount of water to be added

So, for example, to make a 1:5 tincture of echinacea root using 1 litre of alcohol solution at 80%, the desired strength of 45% is achieved by applying the following calculation:

1 litre x (80 ÷ 45)
1 x 1.77 = 1.77 litres

Therefore, to dilute 1 litre of 80% ABV spirit to achieve 45% ABV spirit you will need to add:
1.77 litre – 1 litre = 0.77 litres of distilled water.

Keeping Accurate Records

If you are planning to experiment with different amounts and different types of tinctures and mixtures, accurate record-keeping is essential. It will enable you to keep track of your successes and repeat them, and to avoid repeated failures.

Generally, tinctures are recorded using a ratio of weight of herb in grams to liquid in litres and the percentage of alcohol. For example, a tincture of *Echinacea purpurea* with 1kg of echinacea to 4 litres of alcohol solution at 25% ABV would be recorded as: 25% ABV 1:4.

You should not only clearly label your tinctures themselves but also keep a separate written record. Below is an example of a simple table that can be used to do this.

Name of herb	*Echinacea purpurea*
Source	Own garden
Fresh/dried	Dried
Weight	200g
Amount of alcohol and % ABV	0.5l 80% ABV
Amount of water	0.5l
Final ABV %	40%
Ratio	1:5
Date and batch no.	25/5/20, 001

Making Herbal Syrups

Herbal syrups are made by adding herbal infusions or decoctions to a simple syrup, which consists of sugar dissolved in boiling water. The process preserves and improves the taste of the herbs and is perfect for counteracting some of the bitter flavours that can be a feature of herbal tinctures. Sugar works as a preservative in much the same way as salt, by exploiting osmosis (the natural movement from a lower concentration of solute to a higher concentration across a semi-permeable membrane such as a cell wall). Most bacteria have evolved in an environment with a low sugar concentration, so, when they are placed in a high-sugar solution, the liquid within their cells will be drawn out by osmosis and killed off.

Herbal syrups stored correctly in an airtight container that has been carefully cleaned before use should last for up to a year.

The method for producing home-made herbal syrups is a simple one:

Equipment

Clean airtight jars (preferably dark-coloured glass, as this will extend the shelf life further)
A medium cooking pan
Kitchen sieve
Muslin cloth
A funnel

Method

First, you will need make an infusion or a decoction. The method that you choose will depend on the part of the plant being used. If you are using a delicate flower of leaf, it will need to be an infusion but, if you are using roots, dried berries, bark or tougher plant material, then it will be a decoction.

Infusion

1. Add the herbs to water in an appropriately sized pan, following the simple ratio of one teaspoon of herbs to one cup of water.

2. Bring the mixture to the boil and turn down to a simmer. Simmer for 10–15 minutes or until the mixture has roughly halved in volume.

3. Strain the mixture through a kitchen sieve with a square of muslin cloth placed across it, and decant into a clean jar. This can be kept in the fridge for up to two days but is best used straight away.

Decoction

Follow the same steps as above, but simmer for longer at a lower temperature – at least 20–30 minutes, or until the mixture has reduced in volume by approximately half.

To Make the Syrup

1. To turn a decoction or infusion into a syrup, you will need to add one cup of sugar per 1 pint of your decoction or infusion.

2. Place in a medium-sized pan on to a low heat and simmer for a further 20–30 minutes, until the mixture starts to thicken into a syrup. It is important to keep an eye on the mixture and take it off the heat when the sugar has fully dissolved and the liquid has thickened. Otherwise, there is a risk of burning the sugar and spoiling the flavour of the syrup.

3. Using a funnel, carefully pour the syrup into a dark glass bottle that has been thoroughly cleaned.

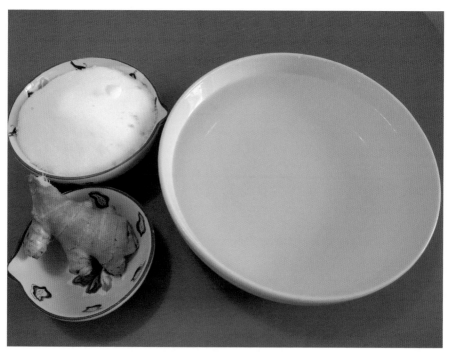

Ingredients for the syrup: ginger, sugar and water.

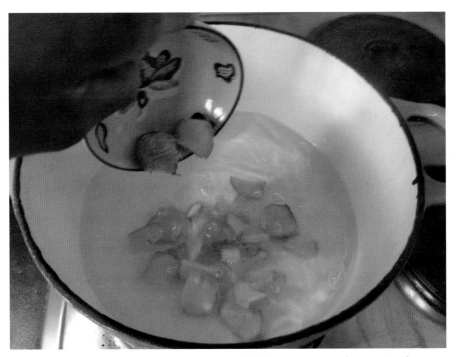

Add the ginger and water to the pan.

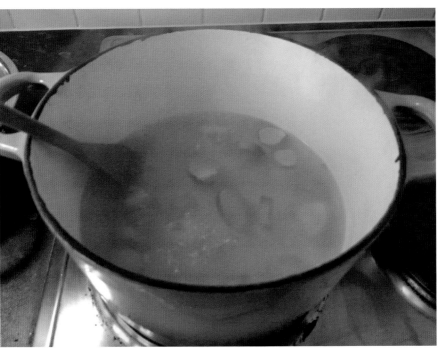

Simmer on the hob.

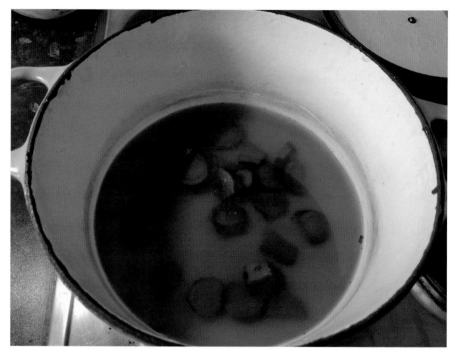

Simmer until the volume is reduced by half.

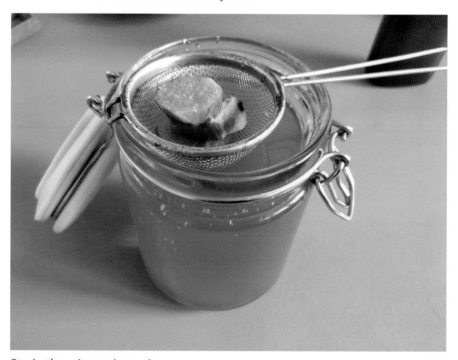

Strain the mixture into a jar.

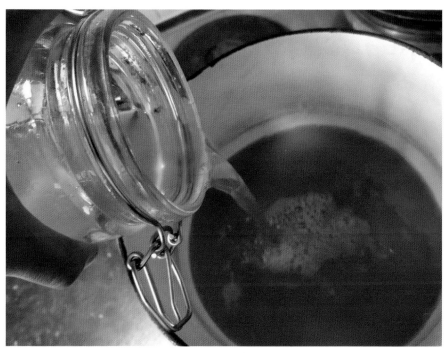

Add the strained mixture back to the pan.

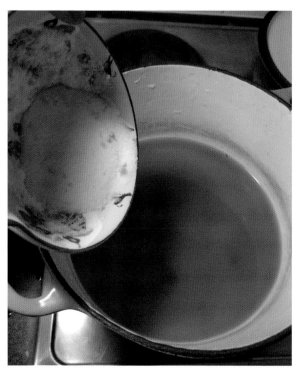

Add extra sugar to the concentrate.

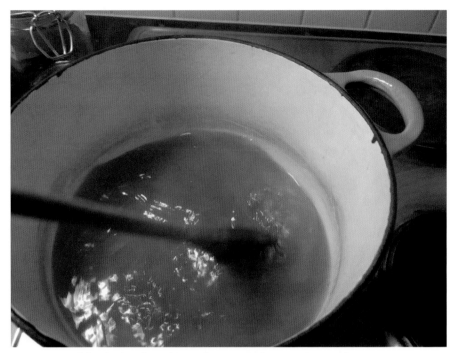

Simmer until further reduced in volume, stirring continuously.

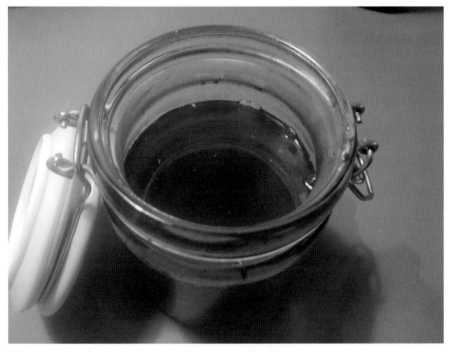

When it is ready, pour the syrup into a sterilized jar.

6

Herbal Elixir Recipes

Principles of Herbal Medicine

Viewing the human body as a complex integrated system rather than as a collection of isolated parts is central to the practice and theory of herbal medicine. This vision of the body is also the driving force behind the use of herbal elixirs, all of which feature a selection of herbs that act upon specific bodily systems or functions in a far wider way than shop-bought pharmaceuticals. For example, if you are experiencing digestive troubles such as heartburn or acid reflux, there are any number of medicines or pharmaceutical products that will treat specific symptoms. In contrast, the approach of the herbalist is to create a mixture of herbal tonics that are designed to strengthen the health and resilience of the whole of the digestive system, rather than addressing a particular chronic disorder alone.

It is important to remember that the body is constantly at work monitoring its external and internal conditions and regulating itself in order to maintain the delicate balance that is vital for health and well-being. It is not unlike juggling and riding a unicycle whilst also trying to hold down a desk job, all at the same time! The chances of making a mistake – of dropping a juggling ball, falling off your unicycle, or forgetting to reply to an important email – greatly increase with thirst or hunger. Herbal tinctures can keep all of the body's systems well fed and watered, so that it can keep on juggling and unicycling without making the sort of mistakes that lead to ill health.

Making Elixirs Delicious as well as Effective

Herbal medicines are most effective when taken regularly but, unfortunately, the taste of many herbal remedies can be off-putting. It is far better to create an elixir

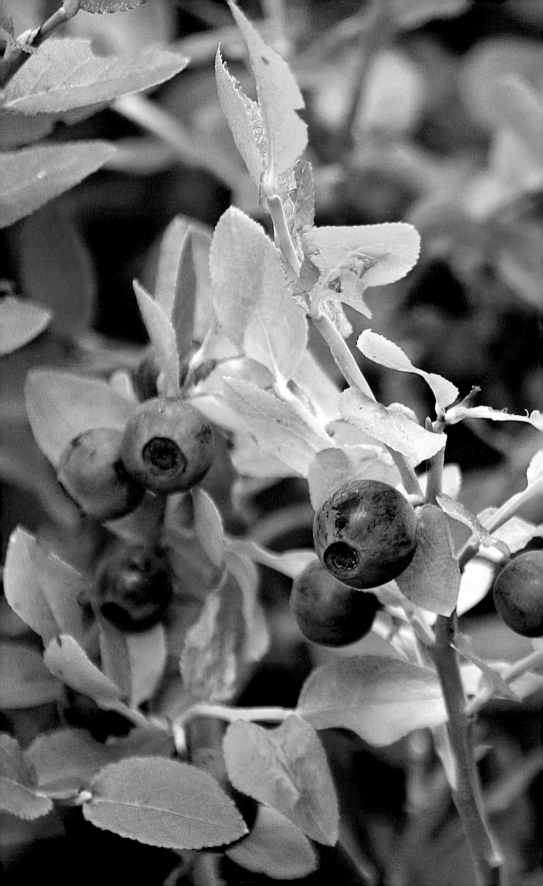

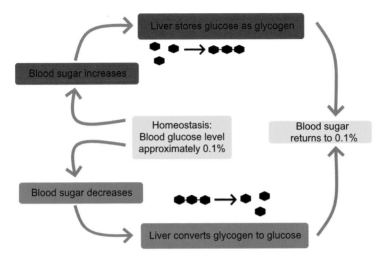

Diagram showing how the body regulates blood sugar to a safe level.

that people look forward to drinking, rather than viewing it as an unpleasant concoction that has to be drunk only *for their own good*.

Many herbal tinctures have a strong bitter taste. Of all the four main taste types – sweet, sour, salty, and bitter – the latter will, for many people, rank as the least favourite. Different tastes can invoke different reactions and have different associations. Whilst sweetness is usually associated with pleasure, and is an indication that a plant is good to eat, bitterness can be perceived as a warning that a plant is not safe to eat. Indeed, many naturalists and foragers recommend nibbling a tiny portion of a wild plant to determine, through taste, whether or not it is edible. Arguably, the distaste for bitter flavours has grown in recent years, as manufacturers have increased the amount of sugar in 'fast' and processed foods. As certain cultures have been drawn more to a taste for the sweet things in life, so their appreciation of more bitter flavours has declined. However, cultural influences still play a big role in taste perceptions and

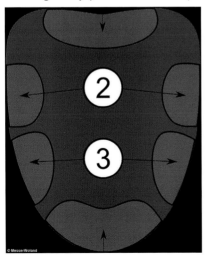

The distinct regions of the tongue that are thought to detect different tastes: 1. Bitterness, 2. Sourness, 3. Salt, 4. Sweetness.

associations, and to this day many Mediterranean countries have maintained a tradition of enjoying bitter-tasting foods and drinks.

Generally, then, increasing the sweetness of an elixir by adding sugar will make it appeal to a wider audience. It is well known that a diet that is high in sugar can lead to a number of health issues, such as an increased risk of diabetes. However, on balance, the benefits of adding relatively small amounts to your elixirs, in order to improve the flavour, will outweigh the negatives.

There is a variety of sugars to be found in any supermarket, but what are the differences between them? In terms of overall sucrose content, refined white sugar and unrefined brown sugar are surprisingly similar. Whilst unrefined sugar will contain more molasses, which can add a richer, more complex flavour, there is no reason not to use refined sugar – it will still do the job! As with the herbs, it is important to use organic sugar, to avoid introducing unwanted chemicals to your product. As the sugar is added for taste alone and does not contribute to or detract from the positive effects of the elixir, you can experiment with amounts, or even remove it all together if you happen to find the natural, unsweetened bitterness enjoyable.

The Recipes

Ingredient Measures

The ingredients in the recipes are given in ratios, or 'parts', rather than in specific amounts. This will allow you easily to make adjustments to suit the volume that you want to produce, from a couple of small jars for the cupboard to a much bigger undertaking. Most home bakers will already be familiar with working with ratios. Each ingredient is specified in a number of 'parts', and each 'part' refers to a consistent amount that remains the same across all the ingredients. The easiest way to make sure your amounts remain consistent is to use one unit of measurement. Luckily, all the ingredients you will be using are liquids, so the simplest approach is to use millilitres, centilitres or litres.

There are two ways you can use the recipes: either designate the amount of your 'part' before you start, or work backwards from a desired total of your end product.

As an example, look at the first method and apply it to the recipe for the immune support elixir. The ingredients list asks for 1 part of echinacea tincture, 1 part of cinnamon tincture, 1 part of ashwagandha tincture, 3 parts of elderberry syrup and 6 parts of a distilled water and alcohol mix. So, if you say that one part is equal to 100cl, the measures you need are 100cl echinacea tincture, 100cl cinnamon, 100cl ashwagandha, 300cl elderberry syrup and 600cl of distilled water and alcohol mix. Of the two methods, this is by far the simplest – ideal if you are not too keen on maths!

For the second method, you decide before on the amount that you would like to produce and work backwards. This method does involve a little mathematics, so eyes straight ahead and try to remain focused! Taking the immune support elixir again as the example, say you want to produce 1 litre, or 100cl, of end product, you can work out the measure of each part by dividing the final total by the number of parts specified in the ingredients list. In this case, there are 12 parts in the list, so you divide 1 litre, or 100cl, by 12. The answer (8.3) is the measure for each one 'part'. From this point on, the process is the same as for the first method. (It can be useful sometimes to convert your measurements – for example, 8.3cl is equal to 83ml – but you must remember to convert across all the ingredients.)

Alcohol Strength

At the Bath Botanical Gin Distillery, all the elixirs are made at around 20% ABV and it is recommended that you aim to do the same. This percentage is strong enough to retain a preservative effect that will allow you to keep your elixirs for up to a year, as long as they are stored out of direct sunlight or in a ceramic bottle. At the same time, it is low enough that the drinks can be enjoyed with, or without, a mixer. It maintains an alcoholic taste that is pleasant when mixed, but not over-powering when consumed on its own.

Determining the exact strength of alcoholic solutions is quite a complicated task, which involves accounting for a number of variables and making a series of complex calculations. You would be forgiven, therefore, if you decide simply to use a 20% distilled water and alcohol mixture, rather than adjusting the percentage of the mixture to account for the alcoholic content of each of the tinctures. However, if you do want to produce an accurate strength, *see* the detailed advice on the process later in this chapter.

Recipe: After Dinner

This elixir is designed to be a sipping drink to be enjoyed after meals. It draws on the European tradition of the digestif.

If indeed 'you are what you eat', as the saying goes, it pays to be aware that you can benefit from what you consume only if your digestive system is able to break down and absorb the nutrients. Research into the gut has revealed a system that is far more complex than it was previously believed to be. It relies on a sur-prisingly large and diverse fauna of bacteria and fungi (known collectively as the microbiome) in order to process food and extract vitamins and minerals that are vital to wider health and vitality.

This recipe contains a mixture of herbs that help soothe and relax the lining of the gastrointestinal system, restoring function and relieving excessive gas, which is often an indication of an irritated gut.

Method
Combine a mixture of your tinctures and distilled water and alcohol mixture in the following ratios:

1 part marshmallow root (*Althaea officinalis radix*)
2 parts peppermint (*Mentha piperita*)
1 part fennel (*Foeniculum vulgare*)
1 part chamomile (*Matricaria recutita flos*)
6 parts alcohol and distilled water mixture

Recipe: Immune Support
This delicious aperitif can be enjoyed straight or mixed with tonic or soda. It is designed to support the immune system.

The key to long-term good health is the prevention of the development of disease and illness. Whilst some experience of ill health is unavoidable, a well-balanced immune system will help your body defend itself against many bacterial and viral infections. Research into the effects of stress have found it to be a major factor in weakening the immune system, so supporting the system is vital in an increasingly stressful world. This elixir uses a blend of echinacea, cinnamon, ashwagandha and elderberry syrup, all of which are known to boost immune health and reduce the symptoms of stress, to have anti-viral properties and to act as powerful antioxidants.

Method
Combine a mixture of your tinctures and distilled water and alcohol mixture in the following ratios:

1 part echinacea (*Echinacea purpurea*)
1 part cinnamon (*Cinnamomum zeylanicum*)
1 part ashwagandha (*Withania somnifera*)
3 parts elderberry syrup (*Sambucus nigra*)
6 parts distilled water and alcohol mix

Recipe: For Aching Joints
This aperitif is designed to be a powerful anti-inflammatory mix. The celery seed gives it a punchy flavour, and it can be enjoyed alone or mixed with tonic or soda. It tastes particularly good mixed with tomato juice.

Health and well-being do not rely solely on functioning bodily systems; they also rely on a functioning body! As the body ages, wear and tear begin to take effect on it, resulting in a build-up of aches and pains. Much of the discomfort is caused by inflammation and irritation of the joints, which develop over time. This elixir uses a mixture of herbs that have been designed to ease inflamed tissue and promote pain-free movement. Chinese foxglove has long been used to treat rheumatism and osteoarthritis, and recent studies have shown it to be useful in aiding bone health and help to protect from bone loss. Native to southern Africa, devil's claw has been used by indigenous peoples for centuries as a natural remedy and cure for a variety of conditions. More recently, studies have found that it can help relieve the pain and stiffness caused by osteoarthritis, particularly when it affects the knee or hip.

Method
Combine a mixture of your tinctures and distilled water and alcohol mixture in the following ratios:

1 part Chinese foxglove (*Rehmannia glutinosa*)
1 part devil's claw (*Harpagophytum procumbens*)
3 parts liquorice root (*Glycyrrhiza glabra*)
1 part celery seed (*Apium graveolens*)
8 parts distilled water and alcohol mixture

Recipe: Menopause Support
This elixir is an aperitif designed to help alleviate some of the negative effects of the menopause, which occurs when the ovaries' production of the hormones progesterone and oestrogen greatly decreases. This can result in a range of issues that vary from person to person but may include depression, sleep problems, joint pain and night sweats. The herbs in this recipe have been shown to have a positive effect on a number of these symptoms. For example, black cohosh, a plant native to North America, has been shown in numerous trials to relieve many of the negative symptoms; sage has been included to reduce hot flushes and night sweats; and milk vetch, a herb commonly used in Chinese medicine, has been included for both its stress-relieving and anti-ageing qualities.

Method
Combine a mixture of your tinctures and distilled water and alcohol mixture in the following ratios:

1 part black cohosh (*Cimicifuga racemosa*)
1 part sage (*Salvia officinalis*)
2 parts liquorice root (*Glycyrrhiza glabra*)
1 part milk vetch (*Astragalus membrosa*)
5 parts distilled water and alcohol mixture

Recipe: Below the Belt

This aperitif has been designed to help address the problems with male sexual function and libido that can sometimes result from the ageing process. Both sexual function and libido rely on a complex interplay of physical and psychological factors. The ingredients comprise a variety of herbs that reduce the physical symptoms of stress, improve the function of those all-important fine blood cells and increase general blood flow around the body. They include, for example, bilberry tincture. Commonly found in mountainous areas all over the world, bilberries are noted for their antioxidant qualities and for their capacity to improve the flexibility of fine blood vessels. Also included are ginseng, which has traditionally been used in Chinese medicine for the treatment of male sexual function, and schisandra, a herb known to improve liver function and reduce inflammation and stress.

Method

Combine a mixture of your tinctures and distilled water and alcohol mixture in the following ratios:

1 part Asian ginseng (*Panax ginseng*)
2 parts *Schisandra chinensis*
2 parts bilberry (*Vaccinium myrtillus*)
4 parts distilled water and alcohol mixture

Recipe: Winter Cold Remedy

This elixir is to be enjoyed as a 'hot toddy', added to a mug of hot water and served with a slice of lemon.

There are many pharmaceutical cold and flu remedies available to purchase over the counter. Whilst there is no doubt that some can be effective, they are primarily designed to suppress the symptoms of illness rather than helping the body to fight off the infection. Having a warm mug of this elixir with a slice of lemon will certainly help you feel a little less sorry for yourself, but the blend of herbs will do more than that – it will also aid your body to battle against the virus. Elderberry has long been used in the treatment of colds and flus and is known for its anti-viral qualities. It is blended here with ginger, which not only tastes good but also has the effect of promoting perspiration, helping the body keep cool while it is feverish, and cinnamon, which has anti-inflammatory properties and also gives a comforting 'Christmassy' taste.

Method
Combine a mixture of your tinctures and distilled water and alcohol mixture in the following ratios:

10 parts elderberry (*Sambucus nigra*)
3 parts cinnamon (*Cinnamomum zeylanicum*)
5 parts ginger (*Zingiber officinale*)
3 parts distilled water and alcohol mixture

Recipe: Lifting the Winter Blues
This aperitif is designed to help lift low mood associated with the changing seasons.

Seasonal affective disorder, aptly shortened to SAD, is a form of illness associated with particular seasons. It is often referred to as 'winter depression' because it is usually more of an issue during the winter months. The main symptoms – low mood and reduced energy levels – can range from mild to severe, but the majority of people living in the northern hemisphere will experience them to some extent.

The blend of herbs in this elixir includes St John's wort, which has a long history of use in the treatment of mental health problems. It contains a number of active substances that are thought to act in a similar way to modern antidepressants, by increasing the activity of certain chemicals in the brain. It is combined here with verbena and ginger, both of which not only taste delicious, but also help to enliven the body and the mind!

Method
Combine a mixture of your tinctures and distilled water and alcohol mixture in the following ratios:

1 part St John's wort (*Hypericum perforatum*)
1 part verbena (*Verbena officinalis*)
2 parts ginger (*Zingiber officinale*)
2 parts distilled water and alcohol mixture

Recipe: Mental Alertness
This may be enjoyed as an aperitif and will help to lift any sense of 'fogginess' in the brain.

Almost everyone will have a time when their thoughts feel sluggish and their memory seems poor. Although it is often associated with the effects of ageing, it can also be brought on by stress and lack of sleep, even in the youngest and most supple of minds. To give your brain a boost, this elixir brings together a mix of herbs that are known to enhance mental capacity. The potent properties of ginkgo leaf have led to its use in the treatment of vascular dementia; Siberian ginseng is known to help relieve stress, fatigue and mental tiredness; and bacopa is used in Ayurvedic medicine to strengthen the memory and improve concentration. Unfortunately, these herbs are particularly strong-tasting, so this elixir does not slip down quite as easily as some of the others. Adding mint syrup can make it fresher and more palatable.

Method
Combine a mixture of your tinctures and distilled water and alcohol mixture in the following ratios:

1 part ginkgo leaves (*Ginkgo biloba*)
1 part Siberian ginseng
1 part bacopa
2 parts mint syrup

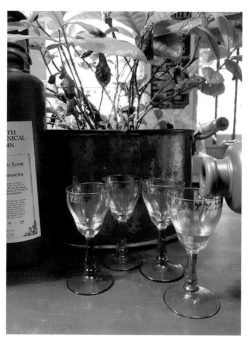

Finally, you should not feel bound by the recipes given here. Be adventurous! You can carry out any number of small-scale experiments on your own, adding syrups instead of tinctures or adding or swapping out herbs. The possibilities are (almost) infinite – just have fun with it!

Serving an after-dinner herbal elixir.

Calculating the Strength of an Elixir

These recipes rely on producing very exact quantities of alcohol within each elixir. As the tinctures contain non-liquids and various different oils, it becomes very hard to get an accurate measure using a hydrometer, as would usually be the case. Instead, to arrive at an accurate ABV you will have to do a series of calculations that take into account the amount and alcohol content of each of the tinctures.

Take the 'After Dinner' recipe as an example, with 1 part being equal to 1 litre:

1 litre marshmallow root tincture @ 25% ABV contains 0.25 litres of alcohol
2 litres mint tincture @ 45% ABV contain 0.9 litres of alcohol
1 litre fennel tincture @ 40% ABV contains 0.4 litres of alcohol
1 litre chamomile tincture @ 40% ABV contains 0.4 litres of alcohol
Total amount of alcohol from tinctures = 0.25 + 0.9 + 0.4 + 0.4 = 1.95 litres

It is now possible to work out how much alcohol needs to be added with the distilled water to make the final elixir at 20% ABV.

Adding 6 litres of distilled water and alcohol mixture gives a total volume of elixir of 11 litres. To be exactly 20% ABV it needs to contain 20% x 11 = 2.2 litres of alcohol.

It already contains 1.95 litres of alcohol from the tinctures so you need to make sure that the distilled water and alcohol mixture contains 2.2 – 1.95 = 0.25 litres of 100% alcohol.

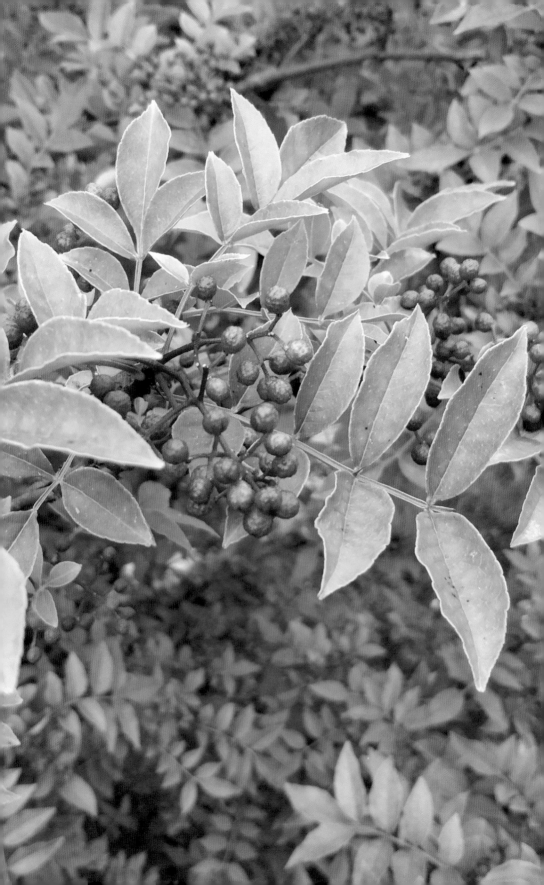

Part 4

Monographs

7

Herbal Monographs

The following list includes botanical information on individual plants, to enable correct identification. It also describes the pharmaceutical properties that can be exploited for medicinal purposes.

APIUM GRAVEOLENS

Common name:
Celery

Key constituents:
Coumarins
Furanocoumarins – bergapten
Flavonoids – apian
Volatile oil – limonene,
    phthalides, beta-selinene

Harvest:
Celery is native to England and Europe and can be found growing both wild and cultivated. The stem can be harvested in late summer to autumn, but it is the seeds that are used in Western herbal medicine. They are best harvested in the autumn.

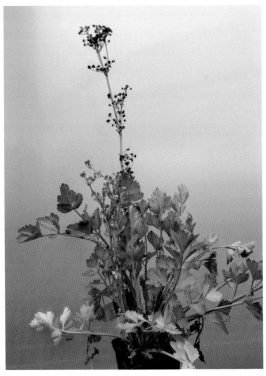
Celery seed (*Apium graveolens*).

Parts used:
Seeds only.

Properties and history:
Celery is best known as a vegetable with a strong and fragrant aniseed flavour, but it has also been used since Roman times in medicinal remedies. The seeds contain apiin, a urinary antiseptic, which has prized diuretic properties. It has been used throughout history as a way of encouraging the body to eliminate toxins through the urine. As a result, the seeds are useful in treating conditions such as urinary tract infections and kidney stones, and to help ease bladder infections. They may also be used for skin conditions associated with poor digestion and liver function, such as acne. Celery seeds are also anti-spasmodic and aid digestion, making them a useful treatment for digestive complaints such as indigestion, heartburn and trapped wind. Their anti-inflammatory effect also makes them an excellent remedy for conditions such as arthritis. The seeds are antimicrobial and have immune-boosting properties, which can help in the beginning of a cold or flu and with respiratory conditions such as asthma. Celery is also beneficial for the female reproductive cycle, and has been used traditionally to bring on periods and to help with lactation. Whilst the stems are a regular part of many diets and often used in smoothies and juices, the seeds are the most effective part of the plant.

Preparation and dosage:
When creating a tincture or decoction with celery seeds, you can use fresh or dried. The stem can be used to make smoothies and juices, or as an ingredient, while the leaves can be used as a garnish. When used in an elixir it can be a very dominant flavour, so be mindful of this when choosing other ingredients. To make a tincture, follow the method in Chapter 5. To make an infusion with the seeds, add 20g of dried fresh root or 30g of dried root to 500ml of hot water, and place a lid over the top. Leave to infuse for 5–10 minutes, then strain and enjoy as a cup of tea.

ALOYSIA CITRODORA

Common name:
Lemon verbena

Harvest:
The leaves are harvested in late summer.

Parts used:
Leaves.

Properties and history:
A deciduous shrub native to South America, lemon verbena grows up to 2 metres tall, with fragrant leaves and pale green flowers. It is often cultivated for its aroma and most commonly used in teas. It was introduced into Europe in the eighteeenth century, when it quickly became a popular drink in the form of an infusion. It is known for its mild sedative qualities and can be helpful for low-level digestive conditions such as excess wind and bloating.

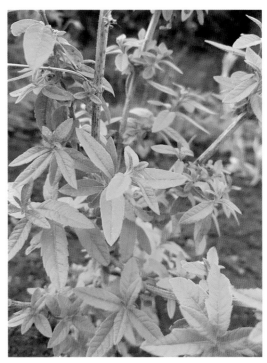

Lemon verbena (*Aloysia citrodora*).

Key constituents:
Volatile oil

Preparation and dosage:
When creating a tincture or decoction, use fresh or dried leaves. When used in an elixir it can add a lovely fresh citrussy flavour. To make a tincture, please see the relevant section. To make an infusion with the leaves, add 5g of fresh leaves or 2g dried leaves to 500ml of hot water, and place a lid over the top, leave to infuse for 5–10 minutes, strain and enjoy as a cup of tea.

Caution:
Lemon verbena is not known to interact with other medicines or negatively affect existing medical conditions.

ASTRAGALUS MEMBRANACEUS

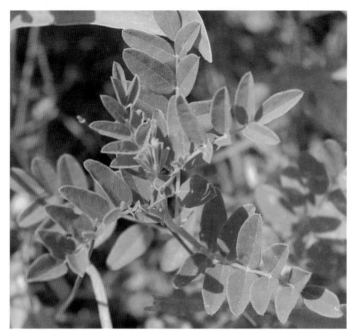

Astragalus *membranaceus* root.

Common names:
Astragalus, milk vetch; also known in Chinese medicine as Huang Qi

Harvest:
Astragalus is a medium-sized perennial that grows wild in Mongolia, and Northern and Eastern China. The underground stem or root is traditionally harvested in the autumn after 4 years of growth.

Parts used:
Rhizome – the part of the stem that grows underground

Key constituents:
Asparagine
Calcyosin
Formononetin
Triterpenoid saponins – astragalosides
Kumatakenin
Sterols

Properties and history:

Astragalus is one of the most renowned plants in Chinese medicine, purported to boost all-round vitality and health mainly through its energizing effect on *wei qi* (said to be an energy or life force under the skin of the body). It is subsequently used interchangeably with ginseng, another herb that is popular for its energizing properties. It is said that this energy can warm the body in colder temperatures and helps to boost immunity to viral infections such as cold and flu. It has also been used in recipes to help with night sweats and hot flushes, due to its action as a vasodilator in promoting blood flow to the surface of the body. Astragalus has also traditionally been used to boost endurance and assist with chronic fatigue conditions. It can also help with digestion, circulatory issues, and may strengthen the urinary system.

Preparation and dosage:

Astragalus will add a sweet, warming flavour to an elixir. To make a tincture from the dried root, follow the method in Chapter 5. To make a decoction, simmer 20g of dried herb or 30g of fresh in 750ml of water for 15 minutes or until reduced to 500ml of liquid, then strain.

Caution:

Do not use if taking immunosuppressive medication, or in acute cases of illness.

CARDUUS MARIANUS

Common name:
Milk thistle

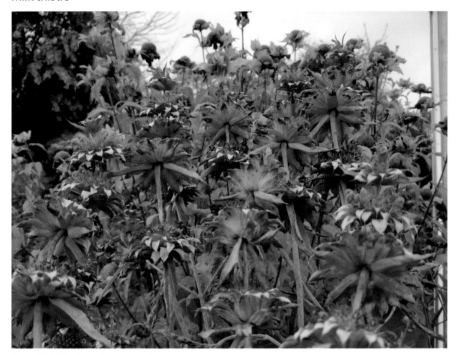

Milk thistle (*Carduus marianus*).

Harvest:
Milk thistle is native to the Mediterranean and now grows abundantly across Europe, North American and Asia, often on waste ground. This biennial can grow up to 1.5 metres tall and has distinctive pink/purple flower heads. The seeds are harvested from the flower head in August/September time.

Parts used:
Seeds.

Key constituents:
Flavonoid – silymarin
Essential oil
Tyramine
Histamine

Gamma linoleic acid (GLA)
Mucilage
Bitters

Properties and history:
Milk thistle has been used for hundreds of years in traditional European herbal medicine. It is renowned for its ability to protect, strengthen and renew and repair damaged liver cells, which is useful for those suffering from conditions that put this organ under stress. These liver-strengthening properties are due to the silymarin that is found in the seeds. Whilst it is the seeds that are most commonly used today, the distinctive white streaked leaves were also used throughout history as a way of promoting the production of breast milk and in cases of depression – in many ancient medicine systems, depression is often linked to poor liver health. As a herb that supports a liver under strain or stress, it is used to help those who consume too much alcohol, and in illnesses such as jaundice and hepatitis. It has also been used to help repair the liver after intensive medical treatment such as chemotherapy. This powerhouse herb is also known to boost the immune system, and to protect the kidneys and therefore assist with urinary issues.

Preparation and dosage:
To make a tincture, follow the method in Chapter 5. To make a decoction of the seeds, simmer 20g of dried herb or 30g of fresh in 750ml of water, for 15 minutes, or until reduced to 500ml of liquid, then strain. Drink half a cup a day for liver infections.

CHAMOMILLA MATRICARIA (ANTHEMIS NOBILIS)

Common name:
Chamomile

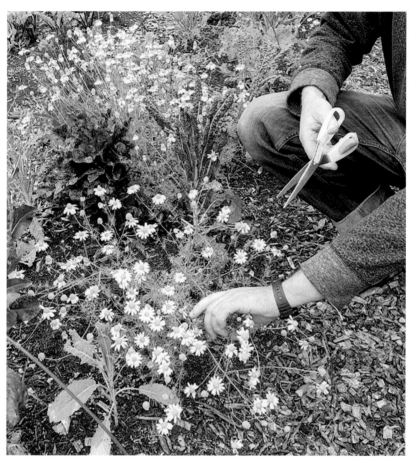

Chamomile flowers.

Harvest:
The yellow and white chamomile flower is a familiar sight, as the plant grows abundantly in the wild across England and Europe. Pick the flower heads in the summer.

Parts used:
Flower heads only.

Key constituents:

Volatile oil – proazulenes, faresine, alpha-bisbolol, spiroether

Flavonoids – anthemidin, luteolin, rutin

Bitters – anthemic acid

Coumarins

Tannins

Properties and history:

This herb can be found in many kitchen cupboards in the form of teabags. It is floral and distinctive, with a slightly bitter taste, and is well known for its sedative and calming properties. Chamomile is the ideal herb to aid restful sleep and soothe a tension headache. It is also brilliant for easing digestive issues linked to stress and emotional imbalance. It is a go-to for those suffering from viral infections, first to soothe fever and infection, and second to boost immunity. It has also been used throughout history to ease period pain, symptoms of PMS and other issues related to the female reproductive system, due to its anti-spasmodic properties. It is also thought to help with conditions such as hayfever and mild asthma.

Preparation and dosage:

To make a tincture, follow the method in Chapter 5. To make an infusion with the flower heads, add 20g of dried fresh root or 30g of dried root to 500ml of hot water, and place a lid over the top. Leave to infuse for 5–10 minutes, then strain and enjoy as a cup of tea. When making an elixir, chamomile will add a sweet, floral and slightly hay-like flavour, and will work best in drinks for relaxation, bedtime and digestion.

CIMICIFUGA RACEMOSA

Common name:

Black cohosh

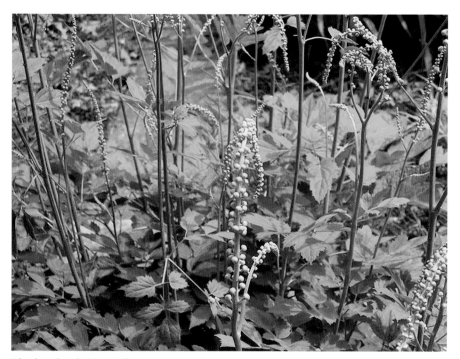

Black cohosh (*Cimicifuga racemose*).

Parts used:

Roots and rhizomes.

Key constituents:

Resin

Bitter glycosides – actein, cimicifugoside

Ranunculin

Salicylic acid

Tannins

Oestrogenic principles

Isoflavones

Isoferulic acid

Properties and history:

Black cohosh is a native American herb used primarily to support and relieve symptoms of each stage of a woman's reproductive cycle. Its oestrogenic properties have the effect of decreasing the ovaries' production of progesterone. It has become the go-to herb for those experiencing hot flushes, anxiety, depression, headaches, and low libido during the menopause. It is also great for balancing hormones in those with high progesterone levels, for regulating the menstrual system for those with excessive bleeding, and for relieving the symptoms of PMS. It is also useful in rheumatic inflammatory conditions such as arthritis. It is a relaxing nervine, which can help those suffering from stress and anxiety.

Preparation and dosage:

To make a tincture, follow the method in Chapter 5. For a decoction, simmer 20g of dried fresh root or 30g of dried root in 750ml of water, for 15 minutes, or until reduced to 500ml of liquid, then strain to enjoy as a tea.

CINNAMOMUM VERUM, CINNAMOMUM ZELANICUM

Common name:

Cinnamon

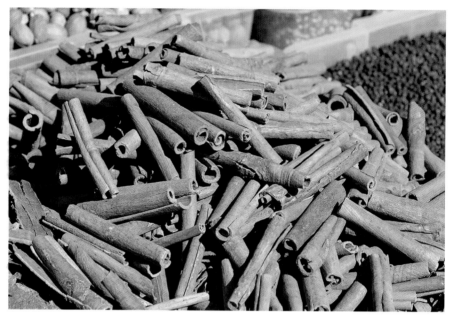

Cinnamon bark (*Cinnamomum zeylancium*).

Harvest:

The evergreen cinnamon tree grows wild in forests in Sri Lanka and India, and various species are cultivated in tropical countries for commercial use. The inner bark is harvested from the new young shoots, and then processed by beating and drying.

Key constituents:

Volatile oils – cinnamaldehyde, eugenol

Tannins

Coumarins

Mucilage

Properties and history:

Cinnamon has been used throughout history as a digestive remedy and holds an important status in Ayurvedic medicine. There is a high percentage of volatile oils (cinnamaldehyde and eugenol) in cinnamon, which have strong anti-viral properties. As such, it is an amazing remedy for infections such as cold and flu, as well as helping to ease fevers, chest infections and dry coughs. It is mildly astringent and helps to stimulate the digestive system, easing conditions of diarrhoea, nausea and wind, as well as conditions such as thrush and candida. The plant also has antiseptic qualities, which help with urinary tract and bladder infections. It may also lower stress and improve mood and low spirits. Cinnamon also contains magnesium, which in conjunction with calcium can help with bone density and muscle stiffness.

Preparation and dosage:
To make a tincture, follow the method in Chapter 5. To make an infusion with cinnamon powder or sticks, add 20g of dried fresh bark or powder or 30g of dried bark or powder to 500ml of hot water. Place a lid over the top, leave to infuse for 5–10 minutes, strain and enjoy as a cup of tea. Its sweet, fragrant flavour makes it ideal for adding to warming cold and flu elixirs, and to digestive elixirs, where its flavour and its digestive and anti-viral properties will be highly beneficial.

Caution:
Do not use in pregnancy or in large quantities.

ECHINACEA PURPUREA, ECHINACEA ANGUSTIFOLIA

Common name:
Purple coneflower

Harvest:
Echinacea is native to North America, but it is widely cultivated in England in private gardens and specialized herb and plant nurseries. The roots should be harvested in autumn, and the cone-shaped flower when it is in full bloom in the summer. This easily recognizable perennial has distinctive purple flowers with a light furry surface and a red-brown central cone.

Parts used:
Roots and sometimes the flowers.

Key constituents:
Alkamides – isobutylamides
Caffeic acid esters – ethinacoside, cynarin
Polysaccharides
Volatile oil – humulene
Echinolone
Betaine

Properties and history:
Echinacea is a popular herb in Western herbal medicine, due to its antimicrobial, antibiotic and anti-fungal properties. It is widely heralded for its strengthening effect on the immune system, helping the body to defend itself against viral and bacterial infections. It will boost the immune system of those recovering from an intense bout of infections and can have a long-term antibiotic use. It is an excellent herb to take on the onset of an infection or at the start of a cold or flu. It has also been used throughout history to help clear skin conditions, such as acne and abscesses, and chilblains, and to ease the inflammatory effects of allergies such as asthma and eczema. It also aids in reproduction infections such as urinary infections and candida, as well as respiratory conditions such as respiratory tract and chest infections, coughs and tonsillitis.

Preparation and dosage:
To make a tincture, follow the method in Chapter 5. To make a decoction, simmer 20g of dried fresh root or 30g of dried root in 750ml of water, for 15 minutes, or

until reduced to 500ml, and strain. For throat infections, try gargling up to three times per day or enjoy one cup per day as a tea. Be aware that the best-quality echinacea tincture should leave a tingly feeling on the tongue.

ELEUTHEROCOCCUS SENTICOSA

Common name:
Siberian ginseng

Harvest:
This powerful herb – not to be confused with Asian ginseng (*Panax ginseng*) – grows wild in Russia, China, Korea and Japan. The root is best picked in autumn and dried before use.

Parts used:
Root only.

Key constituents:
Eleutherosides
Phenylpropanoids
Polysaccharides
Triterpenoid saponins
Glycans

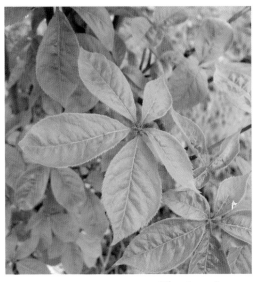

Siberian ginseng
(*Eleutherococcus senticosa*).

Properties and history:
Siberian ginseng has been used in Chinese medicine for over 2000 years. Whilst most herbs are used to treat a specific concern, Siberian ginseng has tradition-ally been used as an adaptogenic herb – a herb that helps the body to cope with exhaustion or stress, both physical and mental, rather than addressing a specific illness or condition. It is useful for situations when a person is under a significant amount of emotional and physical stress, or experiencing feelings of depression. It is also traditionally used for boosting digestion, and is believed to help with diarrhoea, bloating and gas as well as increasing the absorption of nutrients. Its energizing properties have led to its use by athletes, to increase stamina. It may also help cells to dispose of lactic acid, which can ease muscle cramps and sore-ness, as well as boosting the body's natural immune system and recovery.

Preparation and dosage:

To make a tincture, follow the method in Chapter 5. Make a decoction with the root by simmering 20g of dried fresh root or 30g of dried root in 750ml of water, for 15 minutes, or until reduced to 500ml, then and strain and enjoy as a tea.

Caution:

Do not use Siberian ginseng for more than 6 weeks at a time, or at the same time as drinking caffeine.

FILIPENDULA ULMARIA

Common name:

Meadowsweet

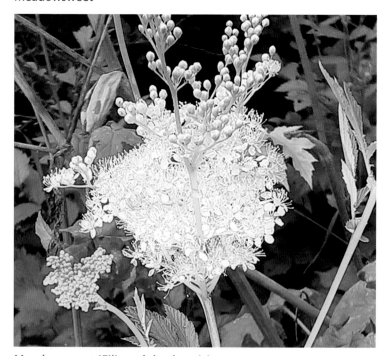

Meadowsweet (*Filipendula ulmaria*).

Harvest:

Meadowsweet can be found growing on riverbanks and in damp grassland elsewhere. The flowers and the leaves are the only parts that should be harvested. The small clusters of creamy white flowers have a distinctive almond smell. Once picked, dry the flowers for future use.

Parts used:

Flowers and leaves.

Properties and history:

The white flowers of meadowsweet adorn the banks of rivers and streams across Europe. The plant grows well in the wild, particularly in damp places. Part of the Salicylate family, it contains an aspirin-like substance (similar to white willow), which makes it an excellent anti-inflammatory herb. As a result, it has been used throughout history as a herbal remedy for arthritis. It is believed that its capacity to neutralize acidity in the body may be one of the reasons why it can help with joint problems. It is also a very good herb for indigestion, as it neutralizes stomach acid. It may also be beneficial for those with IBS, in combination with other herbs.

Preparation and dosage:

To make a tincture, follow the method in Chapter 5. The fresh leaves and flowers make a great infusion: add 30g of leaves to 500ml of hot water, place a lid over the top, leave to infuse for 5–10 minutes, then strain. Drink a small cup of the tea after dinner to help with digestion.

Caution:

Should not be used by those with an allergy to aspirin, or by anyone taking asthma medication, or any medication that interacts badly with aspirin.

FOENICULUM VULGARE

Common name:

Fennel

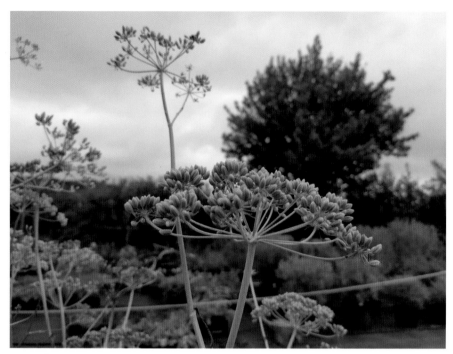

Fennel (*Foeniculum vulgare*).

Harvest:

Whilst fennel is native to the Mediterranean, it is now grown around the world. The seeds, leaves and root can all be harvested, but it is the seeds (collected in the autumn) that are most commonly used.

Parts used:

Seed, leaf, root.

Key constituents:

Essential oil

Phenolic acids

Flavonoids

Coumarins

Furanocoumarins

Properties and history:
It is the benefits of the volatile oils in fennel that make it the go-to herb for digestive issues. It can help with the absorption of vitamins and minerals and is useful for digestive problems such as trapped wind, bloating, stomach pain, nausea, indigestion and heartburn. It is also a great diuretic, helping in the elimination of toxins from the body. Its anti-spasmodic properties help with issues of the reproductive system, including symptoms of PMS and period pains. The plant's anti-inflammatory properties can be beneficial for those with arthritis, and also make it a great herb to use to tackle colds and flu. As a decongestant, it can loosen mucus in chesty coughs and it is also good for those with asthma. As it is mildly oestrogenic, it can benefit the female reproductive system, regulating the menstrual cycle, lessening pain from cramps and PMS, and helping with low libido and menopause symptoms.

Preparation and dosage:
To make a tincture, follow the method in Chapter 5. To make an infusion with the seeds, add 30g of seeds to 500ml of hot water, place a lid over the top, and leave to infuse for 5–10 minutes. Strain and enjoy as a cup of tea. Fennel is known for its sweet aniseed flavour, which adds a pleasant taste to elixirs, and will work best with other digestion-stimulating herbs.

Caution:
Avoid using during pregnancy. Do not use in excess.

GINKGO BILOBA

Common names:
Ginkgo; Bai Guo in Chinese medicine

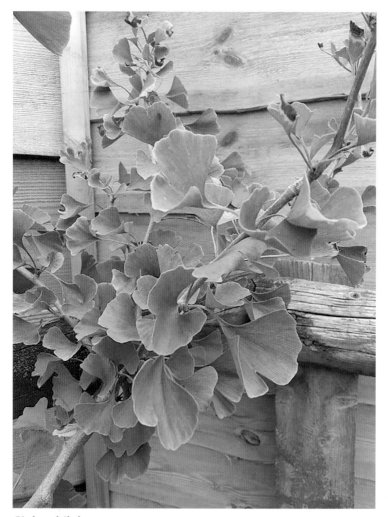

Ginkgo biloba.

Harvest:
Ginkgo trees are native to China, and its fan-shaped leaves are a central part of traditional herbal medicine. The leaves and seeds are harvested at the end of summer and beginning of August.

Parts used:
Leaves and seeds.

Key constituents:
Flavonoids
Ginkgolides
Bilobalides

Properties and history:
The distinctive leaves of the ginkgo tree are not only beautiful but also offer incredible versatility in terms of herbal medicine. Native to China, the trees can reach heights of up to 50 metres and are robust and long-lived, with some thought to be around 2,500 years old. They are thought to be one of the oldest species of tree in the world, appearing in the fossil records of the Jurassic period. The leaves and seeds of the ginkgo tree have long been used in Chinese herbal medicine to treat a variety of conditions, from respiratory problems such as asthma and excess phlegm, to problematic vaginal discharge and incontinence. Products containing ginkgo are popular right across Europe. They are taken by many people from middle age onwards, with a view to improving cerebral circulation and memory, reducing the possibility of stroke and easing the symptoms of senile dementia.

Preparation and dosage:
The leaves are best collected in the autumn when they have turned bright yellow. They have a bitter slightly earthy flavour. To make a tincture, see the relevant section. To make an infusion with the leaves, add 3g of leaves to 500ml of hot water, and place a lid over the top. Leave to infuse for 5–10 minutes and then strain.

Caution:
Avoid taking with anticoagulant drugs.

GLYCYRRHIZA GLABRA

Common name:

Liquorice

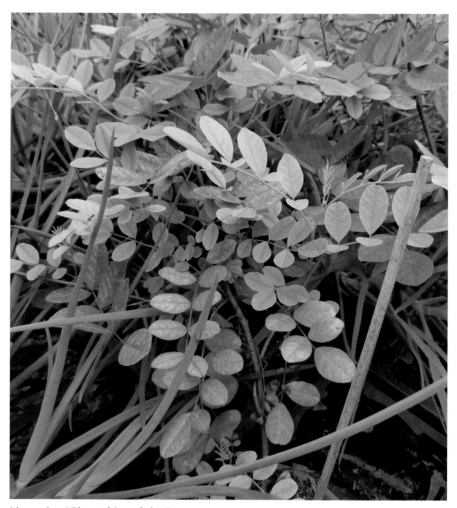

Liquorice (*Glycyrrhiza glabra*).

Harvest:

Liquorice is native to Europe, Asia and North and South America. It is cultivated around the world, and can be found in the UK in specialist herb and plant nurseries. It has been used throughout Europe and the rest of the world for thousands of years.

Parts used:
Root only.

Key constituents:
Triterpene saponins – glycyrrhizin
Flavonoids
Polysaccharides
Sterols
Coumarins
Asparagin
Volatile oils
Tannins

Properties and history:
The root of liquorice has anti-inflammatory properties, along with a super sweet aniseed flavour, thanks to a high percentage of glycyrrhizic acid. It has been used in European herbal medicine to treat a wide range of ailments, and also as a spice to flavour food. In its dried form, the root can be chewed between the teeth for a huge whack of natural sweetness, but also to soothe mouth ulcers. Liquorice is the ideal herb to use to treat digestive ailments such as gastric conditions and stomach ulcers, and can help lower stomach acid to relieve heartburn and indigestion. It also acts as a mild laxative. Its slightly oestrogenic properties can be beneficial for easing menstrual problems, and issues relating to hormonal changes in women, such as the menopause. Liquorice also helps with respiratory conditions such as asthma and chest infections, soothes sore throats and eases dry coughs, and can be beneficial in dealing with inflamed conditions such as arthritis, acne and eczema.

Preparation and dosage:
Liquorice makes an excellent addition to herbal elixirs, not just for its medicinal properties but also for its wonderfully sweet taste, which derives from the glycyrrhizin acid present in the root. It is also used in Chinese medicine to help harmonize the effects when a variety of herbs is used in conjunction. To make a tincture, follow the method in Chapter 5. To make a decoction of the root, simmer 20g of dried fresh root or 30g of dried root in 750ml of water, for 15 minutes, or until reduced to 500ml, then strain to enjoy as a tea.

HARPAGOPHYTUM PROCUMBENS

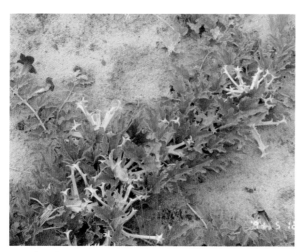

Common name:
Devil's claw

Harvest:
Devil's claw is native to Africa, and grows well on waste ground. It is the roots that are used.

Parts used:
Tubers (roots) only.

Devil's claw (*Harpagophytum procumbens*).

Key constituents:
Iridoid glycosides
Stachyose sugars
Phytosterols
Flavonoids
Harpagoquinone

Properties and history:
Devil's claw has been used throughout history in Africa to treat digestive issues. It is believed that the root, which has a strong bitter flavour, stimulates the digestion and aids with the absorption of nutrients. Devil's claw helps with bloating and constipation, and increases the appetite. It also helps with circulatory problems and can lower heart rate and blood pressure. Thanks to the tuber's anti-inflammatory properties, it is also beneficial for conditions such as arthritis, back pain and rheumatoid arthritis. This could be due to the plant's action on the digestive system and the presence of harpagoside, which reduces inflammation.

Preparation and dosage:
To make a tincture, follow the method in Chapter 5. Make a decoction with the root by simmering 20g of dried fresh root or 30g of dried root in 750ml of water, for 15 minutes, or until reduced to 500ml of liquid, then strain to enjoy as a tea.

HYPERICUM PERFORATUM

Common name:
St John's wort

Harvest:
Flowering around the time of the summer solstice in the northern hemisphere and commonly seen growing wild right across Europe, St John's wort should be collected when it is in flower, and dried immediately.

Parts used:
Flower tops only.

Key constituents:
Volatile oil
Hypericin
Flavonoids
Hyperforins

Properties and history:
This perennial plant grows up to 80cm and is crowned with flat-topped clusters of vibrant yellow flowers. It was considered to have magical properties in medieval Europe and was used to treat emotional and psychological problems. It has strong anti-viral attributes and, when applied externally, can help speed the healing of wounds and prevent infection. However, it is best known for the treatment of nervous conditions, in particular the depression that can result from the changing of seasons (seasonal affective disorder, or SAD) and low moods that are associated with the menopause.

Preparation and dosage:
To make a tincture, see the relevant section. Make a decoction with the flowers by simmering 2g of dried fresh herb or 30g 750ml of water for 15 minutes, or until reduced until 500ml of liquid and strain to enjoy as a tea. Externally, a preparation can be made by steeping the flowers in oil. As an addition to herbal elixirs its flavour is not strong, but it produces a beautiful red colour.

Caution:
Avoid taking during pregnancy. St John's wort can also interact negatively with the following medicines: SSRIs, protease inhibitors, theophylline beta-2 agonists and cyclosporin.

MENTHA PIPERITA

Common name:
Peppermint

Harvest:
This aromatic hardy plant grows freely in gardens across Europe, North America and Asia. The leaves are best harvested in the UK from early spring to late summer, before flowering.

Parts used:
Leaves only.

Key constituents:
Volatile oil – menthol and menthone
Flavonoids – luteolin and menthoside
Phenolic acids
Triterpenes

Properties and history:
Peppermint is more or less guaranteed to be growing in your garden or in garden very close by. It is beautifully fragrant – when you rub a leaf between your fingers, the volatile oils are easily extracted and a strong refreshing smell is released. These volatile oils, especially menthol, a constituent of the oil, are antibacterial, antiseptic and anti-fungal. It is a powerhouse of a herb. The volatile oils provide the digestive properties with which the plant has become synonymous. It has been used traditionally throughout history to ease both diarrhoea and constipation, to soothe nausea and wind, and relax the digestive muscles. Peppermint has also been used to ease headaches and respiratory conditions.

Preparation and dosage:
To make a tincture, follow the method in Chapter 5. To make a decoction, simmer 30g of dried leaves in 750ml of water for 15 minutes, or until reduced to 500ml of liquid, then strain.

Caution:
Do not give to children under 5.

PANAX GINSENG

Common names:
Ginseng, Asian ginseng

Harvest:
Rarely found in the wild, *Panax ginseng* grows in Russia, China and Korea but is largely cultivated for medicinal use. The root is harvested after 4 years of strong growth.

Key Constituents:
Triterpenoid saponins
   – ginsenosides
Acetylenic compounds
Panaxans
Sesquiterpenes

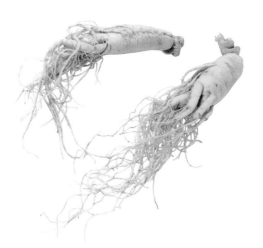

Ginseng (*Panax ginseng*).

Properties and history:
Asian ginseng, not to be confused with Siberian ginseng, is one of the most important and prized herbs in Chinese medicine. It has been used throughout the history of the practice as an adaptogenic herb – one that can help the body's capacity to cope under stress, both physical and mental, rather than addressing a specific illness or concern. The ginsenosides can aid the body in restful sleep and relaxation, but also act to stimulate those lacking in energy. It is commonly used across the world as a male aphrodisiac. Its energizing and relaxation effects make it a popular choice for people who engage in a lot of sports or those undertaking stressful studies or work.

Preparation and dosage:
To make a tincture, follow the method in Chapter 5. To make a decoction with the root, simmer 20g of dried fresh root or 30g of dried root in 750ml of water, for 15 minutes, or until reduced to 500ml of liquid, then strain to enjoy as a tea.

Caution:
Should not be taken for more than 6 weeks and should not be taken excessively or in conjunction with caffeine.

REHMANNIA GLUTINOSA

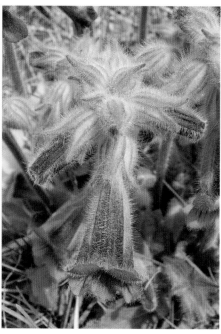

Chinese foxglove (*Rehmania glutinosa*).

Common name:
Chinese foxglove

Harvest:
Native to Northern China, Chinese foxglove can be cultivated from seeds grown in autumn or spring. Harvest the root in the autumn once the flowers have come and gone. The plant is perennial, and grows to 1–2ft, with sticky leaves and purple flowers.

Parts used:
Root only.

Key constituents:
Phytosterols
Mannitol sugars
Rehannin

Properties and history:
This is a long-standing traditional herb in Chinese medicine, known as a 'tonic' herb, due to its tonic action on the liver and kidneys. It had been used traditionally in Chinese medicine to prevent poisoning and liver damage, and it is a popular part of treatment for hepatitis. It is also an excellent herb for lowering blood pressure, for helping with rheumatoid arthritis and for easing the health of the elderly.

Preparation and dosage:
To make a tincture, follow the method in Chapter 5. To make a decoction with the root, simmer 20g of dried fresh root or 30g of dried root in 750ml of water, for 15 minutes, or until reduced to 500ml of liquid, then strain. For the traditional preparation, simmer the same amount of dried root to 750ml of red wine, and reduce to 500ml.

SALIX ALBA

Common name:
White willow

Harvest:
White willow trees are native to Europe, Africa and Asia, but are cultivated to grow in countries with a similar climate.

Parts used:
Bark only.

Key constituents:
Phenolic glycosides – salicylic acid
Flavonoids
Tannins

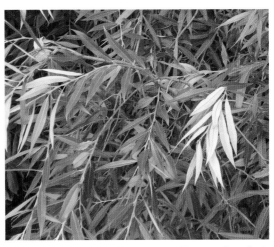
White willow (*Salix alba*).

Properties and history:
White willow has been used throughout history as a natural pain reliever for inflamed, painful joints and for easing the symptoms of fever. It has been referred to as being similar to aspirin, but it does not thin the blood. It does contain salicylic acid, which has the same analgesic and anti-inflammatory effect, and is traditionally used to treat headaches and muscular aches. It is also beneficial in treating issues relating to hormonal changes in women, such as night sweats and hot flushes, and can help ease heavy periods.

Preparation and dosage:
To make a tincture, follow the method in Chapter 5. To make a decoction with the root, simmer 20g of dried fresh root or 30g of dried root in 750ml of water, for 15 minutes, or until reduced to 500ml of liquid, then strain. Drink half a cup three times a day, only when needed.

Caution:
Avoid if allergic to aspirin, and do not use at the same time as taking ibuprofen.

SALVIA OFFICINALIS

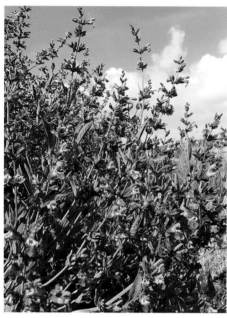

Sage (*Salvia officinalis*).

Common name:
Sage

Harvest:
Sage grows freely in the wild across the Mediterranean, and does well elsewhere in most sunny climates. It is an evergreen plant so leaves are available to be harvested all year round.

Parts used:
Leaves only.

Key constituents:
Volatile oils – thujone
Diterpene bitters
Flavonoids
Phenolic acids
Tannins

Properties and history:
Sage has a wide range of benefits. Because of its antiseptic, antimicrobial and astringent properties, it is widely used in Western herbal medicine for those with colds and flu, sore throats and chest infections. It is also a great herb to use for urinary and bladder infections, and inflammatory joint conditions such as arthritis. It is an excellent aid to digestion, helping with the absorption of fats and with bloating and wind. It helps with a whole host of reproductive concerns, too, especially those related to the menopause, as it can reduce night sweats and insomnia. It can also regulate hormones and painful periods, as it contains phytoestrogens.

Preparation and dosage:
To make a tincture, follow the method in Chapter 5. To make an infusion with the leaves, add 30g of leaves to 500ml of hot water, place a lid over the top, and leave to infuse for 5–10 minutes. Strain and then drink a cup a day as a tea. In an elixir, sage will add a warm, bitter and fragrant flavour.

Caution:
Do not take in pregnancy or when breastfeeding. Do not take if suffering from epilepsy. Do not consume in large amounts.

SAMBUCUS NIGRA

Common name:
Elder

Harvest:
Elder is native to Europe and can be found growing in woods and hedges, and lining parks, canals and gardens. The flowers are harvested from early May, whilst the berries are harvested from August. The flowers are a pale yellow and the berries are a dark purple.

Parts used:
Flowers and berries only.

Properties and history:
Combined with sugar, the flowers of the elder plant create a sweet and floral drink and many people will have made a cordial

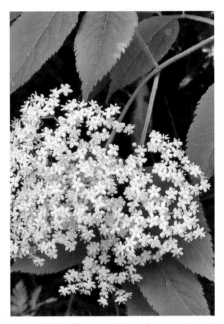

Elderflowers (*Sambucus nigra*).

or a fizz at some point. The flowers can help with hayfever and sinusitis, while the berries have long been used as a traditional remedy for soothing colds, flu and chesty illnesses. Infusions made by simmering the berries in hot water have an effect on cold and flu symptoms by promoting sweating, thereby lowering a fever. Elderberries are rich in vitamin C and are also traditionally used for rheumatism and skin infections. They are also thought to have a mild laxative effect.

Preparation and dosage:
To make a tincture, follow the method in Chapter 5. To make an infusion from the flowers, simmer 20g of flowers in 500ml of water, place a lid over the top, leave to infuse for 5–10 minutes, then strain. To make a decoction from the dried berries, simmer 30g of dried berries in 750ml of water, for 15 minutes, or until reduced to 500ml of liquid, then strain.

Caution:

Take care to remove the flowers and berries from the stems; the stems can be poisonous if consumed in large amounts.

SCHISANDRA CHINENSIS

Common names:

Five-flavour berry, schisandra

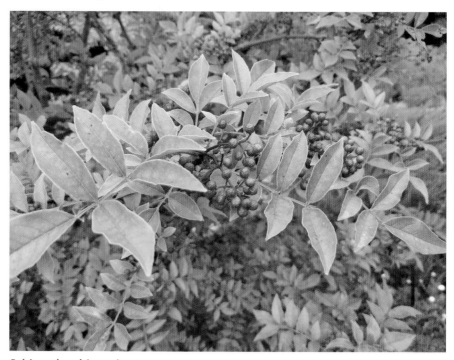

Schisandra chinensis.

Harvest:

Schisandra is native to China, in the north-east. It is an aromatic vine that can grow up to 8 metres, with pink flowers and dark red berries.

Parts used:

Berries only.

Key constituents:

Lignans – shizandrin, deoxyschizandrin, gomisin

Phytosterols – beta-sitsterol, stigmasterol

Volatile oil

Vitamins – C and E

Properties and history:

Schisandra is best known as a traditional Chinese 'tonic' herb, due to its strengthening and toning action on the liver and kidneys, as well as for its stress-relieving properties. It is also known as a 'five-flavoured herb', as it is salty, sweet, sour, spicy and bitter, all at the same time. As a result, in traditional Chinese medicine it is believed to have the capacity to balance all the body's systems. Its traditional use is to ease liver conditions such as hepatitis and poor liver function – the beneficial effects are said to be down to the lignans in the berries. Schisandra is also an adaptogenic herb, helping the body deal with stress, anxiety and insomnia.

Preparation and dosage:

To make a tincture, follow the method in Chapter 5. To make a decoction, simmer 30g of dried berries in 750ml of water for 15 minutes, or until reduced to 500ml of liquid, then strain. Drink 100ml three times a day, but do not drink to excess.

Caution:

Can cause heartburn if taken excessively.

TARAXACUM OFFICINALE

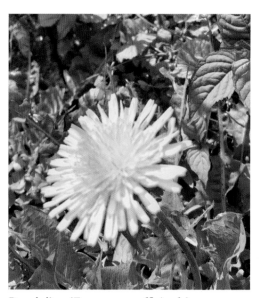

Dandelion (*Taraxacum officinale*).

Common name:
Dandelion

Parts used:
Leaves and roots.

Harvest:
The dandelion plant is native to Europe and Asia and can be found growing wild in England in abundance, where it is seen by most as a weed. The roots are harvested in June and August, when they are at their bitterest. The leaves can be picked at any time of the year, but they should be collected away from roads and fields where pesticides are sprayed.

Key constituents:
Sesquiterpene lactones
Triterpenes
Vitamins – A, B, C
Coumarins
Carotenoids
Minerals – potassium
Taraxacoside
Phenolic acids
Minerals – potassium, calcium

Properties and history:
Dandelion has a distinctive bitter, mineral taste, and has been used in Western medicine predominantly as a diuretic and digestive herb. This vitamin- and mineral-rich plant contains vitamin A, C and B as well as potassium, zinc and manganese. The young, fresh leaves have traditionally been eaten raw or steeped in water to make a tea. Their diuretic effect is useful for treating water retention and urinary tract infections and bloating. The bitter-flavoured roots have

traditionally been used to treat indigestion, conditions such as hepatitis, and skin conditions associated with a build-up of toxins in the liver and kidneys, such as acne and abscesses. The root seems to stimulate bile production in the liver and helps to remove waste products from the liver and gall bladder. The root is also highly anti-inflammatory, making it helpful in conditions such as arthritis and rheumatism.

Preparation and dosage:

To make a tincture, follow the method in Chapter 5. Make a decoction with the roots by simmering 20g of dried fresh root or 30g of dried root in 750ml of water, for 15 minutes, or until reduced to 500ml of liquid, then strain and drink as a tea. Dandelion will add an earthy, slightly bitter flavour to an elixir, so will balance well with something sweet like liquorice. The leaves can also be eaten raw, perhaps added to salads.

VACCINIUM MYRTILLUS

Common name:

Bilberry

Harvest:

Native to Europe and North America, bilberry commonly grows on heathland, moors, and undergrowth on low bushes. The fruit and leaves are collected in the summer. It has oval leaves and small white/pink flowers and dark purple berries, with dark red flesh.

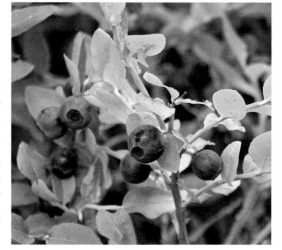

Bilberry (*Vaccinium myrtillus*).
ANNELI SALO/WIKIMEDIA COMMONS

Parts used:

Berries and leaves.

Key constituents:

Flavonoids
Catechins
Invertose

Properties and history:

Bilberries are native to traditional European herbal medicine traditions and have been used for over 1000 years. The berries are best used when they are ripe if being used as a natural laxative, this due to the high fruit sugars. Whilst the dried fruit has an antibacterial effect and is said to be binding, and so is also useful in treating diarrhoea. It is thought the high anthocyanin content makes it useful in treating a wide range of ailments, from cardiovascular conditions, varicose veins, haemorrhoids and to strengthen vision and other ailments related to capillary fragility. The leaves are also traditionally used to treat skin conditions such as scurvy.

Preparation and dosage:

To make a tincture, follow the method in Chapter 5. Steep 20g dried berries or leaves or 30g fresh berries or leaves in 750ml of water and reduce down to 500ml, and strain.

Caution:

Do not use the leaves for more than three weeks.

WITHANIA SOMNIFERA

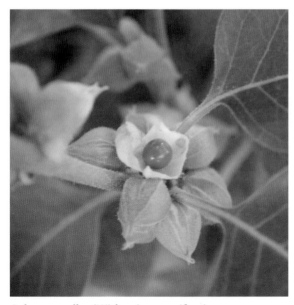

Ashwagandha (*Withania somnifera*).
THAMIZHPPARITHI MAARI/WIKIMEDIA COMMONS

Common name:
Ashwagandha

Harvest:
Withania can be found growing in India, the Mediterranean and the Middle East. The leaves are harvested in the spring, and the root and fruit in the autumn. This hardy shrub has oval leaves with yellow/green flowers.

Parts used:
Root only.

Key constituents:
Alkaloids
Steroidal lactones – withanolides
Iron

Properties and history:
Withania has become synonymous with vitality, life energy and strength, in Ayurvedic medicine, and it is used to ease stress and assist those struggling with 'burn-out' or nervous exhaustion. As with all adaptogenic herbs, withania is really useful for helping the body to cope with long-term stress and the pressure it puts on the body. Because of its energising and reviving effects, it has become known as the 'Indian ginseng'. It is suggested that the alkaloids present in withania are responsible for its ability to lower blood pressure and act as a mild sedative. The withanolides are anti-inflammatory and can help in inflammatory conditions such as rheumatoid arthritis.

Preparation and dosage:
To make a tincture, follow the method in Chapter 5. To make a decoction, simmer 30g of dried berries in 750ml of water for 15 minutes, or until reduced to 500ml of liquid, then strain. Drink 100ml three times a day, but do not drink to excess.

Caution:
Do not consume whilst pregnant.

ZINGIBER OFFICINALE

Common name:
Ginger

Harvest:
This spicy, vibrant root grows well in hot climates and is native to South-East Asia. It has been used in the west for at least 2000 years. It is harvested when the leaves have dried above the ground; these are discarded and only the root is used. The root can be used both dried and fresh.

Parts used:
Rhizome (the parts of the stem that grow underground that appear to be roots).

Key constituents:
Volatile oil – zingiberene
Oleoresin – Gingerol, shogaols

Properties and history:
Ginger root is used to treat a myriad of ailments in traditional Chinese medicine. The ground powder is also a popular spice, which is used to give food an earthy, warming and spicy flavour. Ginger has been used as a digestive remedy to ease conditions such as indigestion, bloating and wind, and its antiseptic qualities also make it a useful plant to use for gastrointestinal infections. It is also prized for its stimulant properties, and has traditionally been used to stimulate circulation, helping with conditions such as high blood pressure, chilblains and fever. Ginger is also a popular diaphoretic for those with colds and flu, as it encourages perspiration, which can bring about a reduction in fever. It contains a high percentage of volatile oils, which can help ease the respiratory symptoms of cold and flu and painful headaches.

Preparation and dosage:
Ginger will add a warming, sweet and spicy element to an elixir. To make a tincture, follow the method in Chapter 5. To make a decoction with the root, simmer 20g of dried fresh root or 30g of dried root in 750ml of water, for 15 minutes, or until reduced to 500ml of liquid, then strain to enjoy as a tea.

Appendix I

Further Reading

Anderson, S. *The Psychobiotic Revolution: Mood, food, and the new science of the gut-brain connection* (Penguin, 2017)

Bone, K. A. *Clinical Guide to Blending Liquid Herbs* (Churchill Livingston, 2003)

Bone, K. and Mills, S. *Principles and Practice of Phytotherapy* (Churchill Livingstone, 2013)

Chevallier, A. *The Encyclopaedia of Medicinal Herbs* (Dorling Kindersley limited, 1996)

De Ruijt, T. *Tonic* (Hardie Grant Books, 2017)

Enders, G. *Gut: The Inside Story of Our Body's Most Underrated Organ* (Scribe Publishers, 2017)

Greger, M. and Stone, G. *How Not to Die* (Flatiron Books, 2015)

Harrar, S. *The Women's Book of Healing Herbs* (Rodale Press, 1999)

Hawkings, K. *Aperitif: A spirited guide to the drinks, history, and culture of the aperitif* (Quadrille Publishing Limited, 2018)

Hoffman, D. *The Holistic Herbal* (Element Books, 1983)

Isted, M. *The Herball's Guide to Botanical Drinks* (The Quarto Group, 2017)

Junger, A. *Clean Gut: The breakthrough plan for eliminating the root cause of disease and revolutionizing your health* (Harper One, 2013)

Mcharry, S. *The Practical Distiller* (Distillery Press, 2010)

McIntyre, A. *The Complete Herbal Tutor* (Octopus Publishing Group Ltd, 2010)

Mills, S. *The Essential Book of Herbal Medicine* (Penguin, 1991)

Pole, S. *A Pukka Life: Finding your path to perfect health* (Quadrille, 2011)

Sterry, P. *British Wildflowers: A photographic guide to every common species* (Collins, 2007)

Tobyn, G., Denham, A. and Whitelegg, M. *The Western Herbal Medicine Tradition.* (Churchill Livingston, 2011)

White, L. and Foster, S. *The Herbal Drugstore: the best natural alternatives to over-the-counter and prescription medicines* (Rodale, 2000)

Wong, J. *Grow Your Own Drugs – A Year with James Wong* (Collins, 2010)

Yong, E. *I Contain Multitudes: the microbes within us and a grander view of life.* (Harper Collins, 2016)

Appendix II

List of Suppliers

GLASS BOTTLES
Ampulla: ampulla.co.uk

Wares of Knutsford: waresofknutsford.co.uk

World of Bottles: world-of-bottles.co.uk/glass-bottles.html

HERBS AND HERBAL PRODUCTS
Avicenna Herbal Products: avicennaherbs.co.uk

Baldwins: baldwins.co.uk/herbs

Fushi: fushi.co.uk

Herbal Apothecary: herbalapothecaryuk.com

Indigo Herbs: indigo-herbs.co.uk

Neals Yard: nealsyardremedies.com/wellbeing/herbal-remedies/dried-herbs

Organic Herb Trading Company: organicherbtrading.com

Rutland Biodynamics: rutlandbio.com

SYRUPS
Bristol Syrup Company: bristolsyrupcompany.com

Pukka Herbs: pukkaherbs.com

BITTERS

The House of Botanicals: doctoradams.co.uk/cocktail-bitters

Bath Botanics Ltd: bathbotanics.co.uk

SPECIALIST HERB GROWERS

Jekka's Herb Farm: jekkas.com

STILLS

Air Stills: stillspirits.com/products/turbo-air-still

Alembic Copper Stills: copper-alembic.com/en

Love Brewing: lovebrewing.co.uk/still-spirits/equipment

Moonshine Stills: Wish Ltd (merchant.wish.com)

Olympic Distillers: olympicdistillers.com

BREWING EQUIPMENT: YEAST, HYDROMETERS, CONTAINERS

Brew Store: brewstore.co.uk/spirits-and-liqueurs/stills-and-distilling-equipment

Cole Parmer scientific instruments: coleparmer.co.uk/c/laboratory-equipment

The Home Brew Shop: the-home-brew-shop.co.uk/acatalog/Still_Equipment.html

USEFUL ORGANIZATIONS

For up-to-date research, to find qualified herbalists and learn more about herbal medicine: National Institute of Medical Herbalists (nimh.org.uk)

For excellent online courses in herbal medicine, from basic to professional level: Heartwood (heartwood-uk.net)

Appendix III

Regulations

Regulations regarding the manufacture of alcohol vary in different countries.

AUSTRALIA

It is illegal to produce alcohol without a licence in Australia, even for personal use. Information is available at: https://www.ato.gov.au/business/excise-on-alcohol/excise-on-spirits-and-other-excisable-beverages.

CANADA

It is not illegal to make a mash in Canada, but distillation needs a licence. For more information:
https://learntomoonshine.com/is-it-illegal-to-make-moonshine-in-canada

NEW ZEALAND

Since 1996 New Zealand is one of the few countries where it is not necessary to have a licence to distil alcohol for personal consumption. You will still need a licence if you want to sell it. Commercial production is subject to tax and licensing as in most countries.

UNITED KINGDOM

In the UK it is not legal to distil alcohol without a licence from Her Majesty's Revenue and Customs. This includes alcohol for personal consumption. Information about how to obtain a distiller's licence is available online from HMRC.

UNITED STATES

US federal law states that it is legal to own a still of any size. However, it is illegal to distil alcohol without having either a Distilled Spirits Permit or a Federal Fuel Alcohol Permit. It does not matter if the alcohol is for personal use only.

Glossary

ABV: an abbreviation of alcohol by volume.

Analgesic: a chemical or substance that has pain-relieving qualities.

Aperitif: an alcoholic drink consumed before a meal to stimulate digestion.

Apothecary: traditionally used to refer to an individual practising medicine, the term now describes a business that sells medicinal products. Similar to a pharmacy but associated with natural and herbal remedies rather than pharmaceuticals.

Autoimmune diseases: conditions in which healthy cells or organs are attacked by the body's own immune system.

Ayurveda: Sanskrit for 'the science of life'; Ayurvedic medicine is the ancient traditional practice of the Indian subcontinent.

Biodynamic: a holistic, organic farming method that evolved from Dr Rudolf Steiner's philosophical and scientific lecturers to farmers. The practice focuses on building up healthy nutritious soil through natural practices such as crop rotation and natural composting instead of using damaging fertilizers.

Botanical: describes a substance derived from plants, usually used as a medicine or flavouring.

Decoction: a method of extracting the water-soluble active constituents of tough and woody plant material into a concentrated liquid. The plant material is added to water and boiled until the liquid reduces by half.

Digestif: an alcoholic drink consumed after a meal to stimulate digestion.

Distillate: a liquid formed through the process of distillation.

Distillation: the technique of heating liquids to boiling point to create a vapor that is then cooled separately from the original liquid. It is based on the different boiling point or volatility values of the liquids. The technique is used to separate components of a mixture or to aid in purification.

Functional food movement: a switch to consuming foods that provide nutrients and nourishment, with the aim of promoting optimal health and targeting and preventing specific illnesses.

Herbal elixir: a medicinal drink made from plant extracts and alcohol, intended to be enjoyed as a drink and also for its medicinal benefits.

Hydrometer: an instrument that measures the density of a liquid. An alcohol hydrometer has been specially calibrated to calculate the strength of alcohol in an alcohol and water mixture. It will not give an accurate measurement if the solution contains other components, such as sugar, which will affect the density.

Infusion: the result of extracting the water-soluble active constituents of fresh and dried delicate plant material such as leaves and flowers. The plant is steeped in water for anything from 15 minutes to 24 hours.

Maceration: the submerging of fresh, frozen or dried fruits or herbs in liquid to soften them. Sugar is often used in conjunction with the liquid, as it draws out moisture. The material being soaked will take on the flavour of the soaking liquid.

Meniscus: the curve on the surface of water when it is in contact with another material.

Menstruum: a substance with the ability to dissolve solids or hold them in suspension. Similar to solvent.

Metabolism: a term that describes all the chemical processes that occur in an organism to keep it alive and functioning.

Metabolite: a substance formed by, or necessary for, metabolism in an organism.

Microbe: a micro-organism that causes disease or the process of fermentation.

Microbiome: the name given to the genetic material of all the microbes – bacteria, fungi, protozoa and viruses – that live on and inside the human body. Often used interchangeably with 'microbiota'.

Microbiota: term that refers strictly speaking only to the organisms of the microbiome and *not* their genetic material. Often used interchangeably with 'microbiome'.

Osmosis: the movement of solvent molecules through a semi-permeable membrane (cell wall).

Phytochemistry: a branch of chemistry concerned with plants and plant products.

Solvent: a term applied to a large number of chemicals and substances that have the ability to dissolve or dilute other substances.

Synergistic interaction: the combination of a number of chemicals, creating an effect that is more beneficial than the effect of each chemical used individually. For example, two herbs used together to target a specific ailment in different but complementary ways.

Tincture: a medicine formed by dissolving herbs in alcohol.

Index

ALSO AVAILABLE FROM CROWOOD

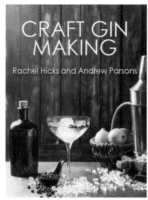

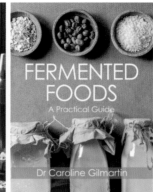

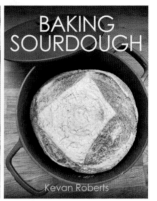